ADVANCE PRAISE FOR *THE TELL*

"*The Tell* is a beautiful account of the journey of courage it takes to face the truth of one's past, and the beneficial role that a combination of skillful therapy and psychedelics can play in putting one's life in order."

—BESSEL VAN DER KOLK, #1 *New York Times* bestselling author of *The Body Keeps the Score*

"Transformative and illuminating . . . Through every agonizing revelation, Amy Griffin refuses to pave over her pain, opting instead to embrace the entirety of it. This is a powerful story of what can happen when self-compassion replaces fear as the governing force of one's life."

—CHANEL MILLER, *New York Times* bestselling author of *Know My Name*

"Amy Griffin has done something remarkable: She's turned life-shattering trauma into a life-giving gift. *The Tell* is the most powerful memoir I've read in years. It's the rare story that will liberate you from shame, empower you to stop cycles of abuse, and make it safer for you to tell the truth. It broke my heart and still left me filled with hope."

—ADAM GRANT, #1 *New York Times* bestselling author of *Hidden Potential*

"Amy Griffin's courageous, generous memoir is both a reckoning with a terrible, all-too-common experience and a searching and empathetic inquiry into the meanings of goodness, self-blame, and forgiveness."

—HANYA YANAGIHARA, *New York Times* bestselling author of *A Little Life* (on Instagram)

"Our minds may repress, but our bodies keep the score. *The Tell* by Amy Griffin is an honest book that will help us trust that wisdom. There is no better guide than Griffin, whose story proves it is what we do with our experience that matters."

—GLORIA STEINEM

"An extraordinary memoir paced like an expertly plotted thriller, each page unraveling the mystery of who Amy Griffin is and what happened to her . . . The moment the truth is revealed stopped my breath in my throat. Griffin's story enraged me, shocked me, broke my heart and put it back together again—I will be thinking about this book for a long time."

—JESSICA KNOLL, *New York Times* bestselling author of *Bright Young Women*

"Overflowing with heart and determination, *The Tell* is the story of a journey—the day-by-day, step-by-step, hard-won push through harrowing emotional terrain. Here is someone moving steadily toward freedom and spreading so much light along the way. In finding the words to tell her story, in showing what it is to trust herself, Amy Griffin shines a path forward through the dark."

—MARISKA HARGITAY

"I started *The Tell* while sitting in my car, after an appointment, and literally spent the morning in the parking lot because I couldn't stop reading. What a generous story. What beautiful writing, crafting, and pacing. And what a heart Amy Griffin has. Your own heart will break, and mend, as you read her story."

—SUSAN CAIN, #1 *New York Times* bestselling author of *Bittersweet* and *Quiet*, and host of the Quiet Life community

"Lyrical . . . though it would sound strange to describe the account of something this dark as 'good,' Griffin has indeed validated her experience with a well-written and moving book. An important, wholly believable account of how long-buried but profoundly formative experiences finally emerge."

—*Kirkus Reviews*

THE
TELL

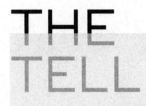

A MEMOIR

AMY GRIFFIN

THE DIAL PRESS · NEW YORK

Copyright © 2025 by Amy Griffin

Published in the United States by The Dial Press, an imprint of Random House, a
division of Penguin Random House LLC, New York.

THE DIAL PRESS is a registered trademark and the colophon is a
trademark of Penguin Random House LLC.

Library of Congress Cataloging-in-Publication Data
Names: Griffin, Amy (Businesswoman), author.
Title: The tell / Amy Griffin.
Description: New York, NY: The Dial Press, [2025]
Identifiers: LCCN 2024035604 (print) | LCCN 2024035605 (ebook) |
ISBN 9780593731208 (hardcover) | ISBN 9780593731215 (ebook)
Subjects: LCSH: Griffin, Amy (Businesswoman)—Mental health. |
Adult child abuse victims—United States—Biography. | Businesswomen—
United States—Biography. | Hallucinogenic drugs—Therapeutic use.
Classification: LCC RC569.5.C55 G75 2025 (print) | LCC RC569.5.C55 (ebook) |
DDC 362.76/4—dc23/eng/20241001
LC record available at https://lccn.loc.gov/2024035604
LC ebook record available at https://lccn.loc.gov/2024035605

Printed in the United States of America on acid-free paper

randomhousebooks.com

9 8 7 6 5 4 3 2 1

First Edition

Book design by Debbie Glasserman

For John

Warning: This book contains depictions of sexual assault. Reader discretion is advised. Please take care of yourself while reading.

There must be those among whom we can sit down and weep, and still be counted as warriors.

—ADRIENNE RICH

CONTENTS

AUTHOR'S NOTE

This is the story of a secret. A secret kept for decades, one I had buried so deep I didn't even know it was there. Many of us carry secrets: things that we were told not to reveal or things we simply couldn't—for fear of judgment or reprisal or, worst of all, for fear that if the people we love found out, they'd see us differently. Sometimes we keep secrets to survive. Then a moment arrives when the usefulness of the secret expires. Keeping it becomes the thing that hurts us. We have to tell.

When I was little, to tell on someone was a shameful thing: It made you a tattletale. It got somebody in trouble. In telling, you became the problem. Now I understand that the telling is the medicine—not the cause of shame but the thing that heals it.

I wrote this book twice. First, for me, painstakingly documenting everything that was happening in real time. The second time, I returned to my initial notes with the distance of all I'd learned in the intervening years. This book incorporates material from my journals, detailed accounts of conversations with family and dear friends, and notes from visits with doctors and other practitioners, as well as scenes reconstructed from memory.

I have spent much of my life as a private person. Like so many women, I have been conditioned not to take up too much space. I was taught to prioritize the comfort of others and not to share anything overly personal. But I have learned that the more I tell my story, the more I remember who I have always been.

By telling you this story, I hope it helps you remember who you are, too.

THE TELL

PROLOGUE

I ran.

    I ran in the mornings and in the afternoons, and I ran at night. I ran on the dirt roads through Palo Duro Canyon, in the Panhandle of Texas, where I grew up, jumping over the cattle guards and dodging rattlesnakes, to the pasture where the horses roamed free. With no one around, I felt free too, like I'd arrived at a place where nobody could touch me. You could see for miles out to the walls of the canyon in the distance. I loved being in motion, and I was proud of the mechanics of my body. The sun would set over the mesa, turning the sky golden, then blue. The fireflies would come out. Bullfrogs croaked in the distance. And I ran.

    I ran at summer camp and around the track at a high school in Oklahoma when I visited my grandparents for Thanksgiving. I ran in college, on the lawn, up the rotunda steps, and in and out of the serpentine garden pathways. I ran in New York City, where I moved after school, along the West Side Highway at night, although I knew it was dangerous. After I was married, I ran in Central Park nearly every morning, while the world was still asleep, dawn just breaking over the tree line. Everyone else who was running in the park at that hour had the same furious intensity as I did. We were the dedicated ones, the ones who would make it out for a run under any circumstances, no matter how hard it was raining or snowing.

I ran when traveling all over the world, never mind the jet lag. In Laos, I passed three monks meditating in a pagoda. Their robes were bright orange, simple, and beautiful. The morning light hit them just so. I thought about them as I ran through the open-air market, past wooden bowls and sewn-cloth bags, wondering what it would feel like to be that peaceful.

I ran in low-ceilinged hotel gyms on old treadmills. I ran on golf courses. "How many loops did you do today?" my dad would ask when I came home for the holidays. It was important to me to know that when I arrived at breakfast on a vacation with my family, I could say: *I already went for a run. I did it.*

Did I enjoy it? I did, on some level, but I never let myself ask that question. Running was just something I had to do, something I had always done. People, sometimes in a vaguely accusatory way, would wonder aloud about my exercise habits. "Do you run so you can eat the chocolate cake?" a friend of a friend asked at a dinner party. She eyed the last bit of whipped cream on my fork as I set it down on my dessert plate. I felt exposed, even though she had misidentified my motivation.

It wasn't about the cake. I always ate the cake.

I ran because I was afraid of what I would feel if I sat still.

I WAS PLAGUED BY injuries; I had surgery on my lower back, then eventually on each of my hips. One rainy afternoon several years ago, I went to see a physical therapist that a friend had recommended to me. I was in a rush, bolting through the city to make it to my appointment on time. My nerves were shot by the time I arrived.

The physical therapist's office was in a fourth-floor walk-up; I could see the elevator was rickety, so I took the stairs, as I often did, since I didn't like confined spaces. As I lay face down on a massage table, the black pleather covered by a thin sheet of exam paper, she pressed her hand onto the left side of my lower back, which made me flinch reflexively.

"It seems like you're doing too much," she said as we spoke about my lifestyle. Her voice was soft and gentle. "Do you always move this fast?"

"I don't know," I said.

"Your body is starting to break down," she said. "I think today we should take it easy. See how your body responds to gentle stretching and stillness."

"No," I said. "I need to move."

I became aware of a heavy, nauseated feeling in my stomach. There was a hollowness in my head, a vague buzzing in my ears.

"You're not listening to yourself," she said. "There's something your body is telling you that you don't want to hear. What is it?"

Suddenly I felt tight, zipped up, locked away. I did not have an answer for her, or if I did, I knew that I could not

put it into words. She was right, of course; there was something. I looked around the room to distract myself. I studied the books on her shelf—had I read any of them? There
was a cup of warm tea steaming beside me, but the air
was cold. Sunlight peeked through the window behind her,
streaking the floor in bars of light. It looked familiar
somehow, like something I'd seen in a dream or a distant
memory.

"Amy?" she said. "Are you all right?" I felt wetness on my
cheeks. I pressed my hands to my face, which was streaked
with tears. She looked concerned. "I'm so sorry," she said. "I
didn't mean to upset you."

"No, I'm sorry," I said. "I don't know why I'm crying. I'm
so embarrassed." I composed myself and thanked her before
heading back out into the bustle of the city. I never went to
see her again. Yet I thought about her for years—what she'd
asked me, and how it must have felt for her to have this
strange woman crying in her space over such an innocuous
question.

She had observed something in me that I could not see
myself. It was like I had a tell—a giveaway, a gesture, the way
poker players do, that indicated I was hiding something.
Mine was my need to push harder, to run faster, to keep
moving. My fear of slowing down long enough to listen to
what my body might say.

She could see that there was something so deep within
me that I did not even know it was there, a presence with no
name or shape. Not an awareness but instead the absence of
awareness. The way it felt to know that there was something
about myself I did not know.

· · ·

WHAT IS IT LIKE to hide something from yourself? Even after all this time, I cannot explain it. We talk about people being in denial as if it were a choice, a voluntary state. Like you can just snap your fingers and it's over, easy as waking up. But it's not like that. Denial is not a switch that can be turned off and on. Denial is a glass case that must be shattered before you realize you were trapped inside it in the first place.

For many years, there were stories I could not tell. Secrets I guarded so tightly that I'd forgotten where I put them. Truths I ran circles around, believing that if I ran fast enough, they wouldn't catch up with me. I know now that this was an act of self-delusion.

The physical therapist had touched a nerve, but she hadn't quite asked the right question.

She'd wondered why I was moving so fast—why I couldn't seem to stop running. For such a long time, people discussed my running. It took up so much space in my life. And yet nobody ever thought to ask:

What are you running from?

I. RUNNING

1. FREE

want to tell you about the things that I remember. The things I have always remembered, things I remember still. The way it felt as a little girl when I'd get on my banana-seat bike, faded pastel pink with tassels on the handlebars, and ride through the streets of Amarillo with the breeze on my face. The sound of the cicadas chirping in the summertime. The way a change in the wind on the cattle yards outside of town, caked with manure, could leave you running for cover. Or a surprise on the cherry tree in our front yard: a loveliness of ladybugs swarming along its bark. I would stand there with a jar, collecting them excitedly. They would crawl up the glass, and I'd watch for a while, naming them. Then I'd set them free.

Free—that was what my childhood in the Texas Panhandle felt like to me. Free like the wide-open spaces, where you could see for miles. Free to stay out until dark, trusting that nothing bad would happen. Free to do cartwheels through the park. Free to roam the neighborhood in search of friends who wanted to ride their bikes to the convenience store for a Coke and a candy bar.

MY FAMILY OWNED THAT convenience store, and several others in town. They were called Toot'n Totum, and there were locations all over Amarillo. The closest to our house was the store on Wimberly. My friends and I would ride there, then use our kickstands to park our bikes next to the building, up against its red-and-white-brick siding, leaving the bikes unlocked.

I can hear it now in my memory: the swish of the door opening and the jingling bell announcing the arrival of a customer. I can feel the blast of air—flat and cold—hitting my face as I walked inside, a reprieve from the dry heat. I can see the hot dogs that had been turning too long in the hot dog machine, which probably needed to be thrown out; my dad didn't like when they were overcooked, which they often were. In the front aisle, there was candy, and lots of it, with a colorful array of gum: I liked the bright, shiny yellow of Juicy Fruit and the synthetic watermelon tang of Hubba Bubba. Chewing gum was discouraged in my family, so much so that my grandmother Novie didn't allow it, considering it an offense as bad as smoking. Once, at a restaurant, my father pointed out a pretty woman smoking a cigarette. "See that woman over there?" he said. "Do you think she's beautiful?"

"Yes," I said.

"No," my dad said. "She'll be wrinkly soon, because she smokes." This was a clever way of keeping me and my siblings away from cigarettes, by appealing to our vanity. Tattoos and motorcycles were similarly verboten, but you couldn't get either of those at the Toot'n Totum.

My favorite snack, the choicest of all options, was a bag of Funyuns. Or I'd mix up a Slush Puppie, pulling the handle to dispense the frozen ice; the store had a machine where you pumped the syrup yourself, and I would use all the flavors, one after another, so that the slush turned my teeth black. Sometimes I would go into the store with my father, usually to pick up a case of Capri Sun when my mom volunteered to bring the drinks to a soccer tournament or community fundraiser. We would walk to the back, into the walk-in freezer where the drinks were stored, past the racks of Hostess Twinkies, Mrs. Baird's white bread, and Planters peanuts. My dad had a sweet tooth: He would usually pick up a pack of M&M's, alternating between classic milk chocolate and peanut; it was always a surprise that I would find stashed, half melted, in the center console of his Suburban. The clerk, in a bright-green apron with pockets, would ring us up, smiling under fluorescent strip lights. When I looked down at my pink jelly sandals, I'd see the gleam of the white linoleum floors, always spotless. Everything was perfect.

Toot'n Totum wasn't the only store in town. Sometimes I would ride my bike to Joan Altman's, a gift shop in a strip mall not far from my house, where there was candy in the shape of red and black berries. I would study them, trying to decide which color I liked better, even though they tasted the same; or did they? I could never tell. Joan had gray hair and a demeanor that could turn on a dime; depending on the day, she would be either delighted to see us or cranky about having her store invaded by a pack of unchaperoned children. My mother went to Joan's to purchase monogrammed gifts. In the South, anything that could be personalized would be—towels and Dopp kits and coasters and mugs, and anything we might need for summer camp. One Christmas I got a turquoise Jon Hart barrel bag with my name stitched on a tan rawhide patch; I can see it in my memory, on the shelf of the closet of my childhood bedroom. The bag was a symbol of possibility—the places I might go, the new people I might meet there. They would know my name because it said it on my bag.

There were two worlds. There was the one outside, where I could be wild, always in a swimsuit, my hair bleached from the summer sun and dry umber dirt under my fingernails. I was as rugged and free as the longhorns that, according to folklore, still roamed Palo Duro Canyon. Then there was the world inside, a world of things, which was ruled by order, exemplified by the stores my family owned. The aisles and shelves were organized, each product perfectly lined up. Space was maximized in the interest of efficiency. Surfaces were tidy. Things were put away where they belonged. Everything was bright, colorful, and ready for purchase.

That order was a form of safety. Life, I thought, would be better if everything could be presented like the items in that store, packaged or frozen. I believed that the things that we sold at my family's stores were good because we sold them. And what we sold—what was good—was convenience. This—convenience—was very important. The best things in life weren't free. They were shrink-wrapped.

When I was little, I loved entertaining my friends at the

store, treating them to feasts of Reese's Pieces, Cool Ranch Doritos, and lemon Gatorade, which I could put on the family account. Eventually, my father had a talk with me. "Amy," he said, "can we talk about the monthly tab?"

"The tab?" I asked.

"From the store on Wimberly," he said. "What do you think happens when you write down what you've bought on that little piece of paper?" I had never thought about it—it seemed more like magic. "I have to pay for all of it," my dad said. It was the first time I understood that everything has a cost.

THE FAMILY BUSINESS WAS only about as old as my father; his parents had opened their first store in Amarillo around the time he was born. At the first location, customers would drive up and honk their horns, and then a clerk would ferry their order out to the car. The store was named for the toot of the car's horn and the toting out of the goods.

Five years after my grandparents started the business, my father's father, whom everyone called Lefty, fell from a ladder while cleaning the gutters. They weren't sure if he'd died of a blood clot or a heart attack; either way, he was gone. My grandmother Novie was widowed with two small children, my father only four years old. But over the next two decades, she expanded the business such that there were nearly thirty locations, a big presence in a small town, by the time I was a little girl. I was the oldest of my parents' children, followed by my brother Jeff, one year my junior. Three years later, my sister, Lizzie, was born, then my youngest brother, Andrew.

Novie's house was as orderly as her stores. The four of us

grandkids bounded like a pack of wolves through her beautiful home in search of dinner rolls or Andes mints. Novie arranged every little decorative object just so. You could feel the tension when we ran through her living room, as if the adults were just waiting for us to topple a potted plant or piece of antique silver. Her house even smelled important somehow, like orange and clove.

Novie had a beloved decorator, a man named Tom, who was frequently at her side, bringing her objects from around the world, like a silver turtle that made a buzzing sound when you pressed down on its tail; she also had a housekeeper who cooked and cleaned. It was novel to me that Novie, a woman, had help with domestic tasks; it meant her hours were free to run her business. It made her life more convenient.

Eventually, Novie found a new partner, Harley, a taciturn man who helped her expand the business; Harley was the only grandfather I ever knew. But no one ever said, "This is your step-grandfather, as your real grandfather is no longer alive." It wasn't until I saw a photo of a young man in a football uniform, standing proudly with his hands on his hips, and I asked who it was, that I understood that this was my paternal grandfather, Lefty, who had been a star athlete before his death.

I began to see that there were things, adult things related to matters of intimacy, that people just didn't talk about. Nobody said that Tom was gay, although it was obvious that he was different from other men I knew, nor did they comment on the fact that Harley and Novie slept in separate bedrooms, as we once discovered when we were playing hide-and-seek in her house. My mother assured us that babies were delivered by stork.

Somehow my grandmother had grown her business into a budding empire as a widowed woman in the South in the 1950s, which was a marvel to me. She had to be tough, and my father was too—handsome, charismatic, and ambitious, to be sure, but also tough. He prided himself on the accomplishments of his children. Even as a very little girl learning to jump rope, I knew I could win his approval through physical trials. A fifty-yard dash. Push-ups. Pull-ups. "How did you compare to the other kids?" he would ask me. Idleness was the devil's work; hard work led to success.

His devotion was as fierce as his expectations were high. The absence in his life that his own father had left behind was vast. He was determined to be present, to never miss so much as a Little League game. He was home every day at five thirty, predictable as clockwork. He coached my softball and soccer teams in the park down the block. He had no playbook on how to be a father, because fatherhood had never been modeled for him. Yet somehow he figured it out in real time, never letting us see him sweat.

From my father, I learned what it meant to be a businessperson. I understood that his employees at the family business, where he came to work after he graduated from college, were a community that needed to see his leadership. On weekends and holidays, he would drive around and check in on the clerks to make sure business was running smoothly, then come home with a box of hot doughnuts from the Donut Stop, including a cherry glazed that, once I'd eaten it, made me look like I was wearing bright-red lipstick—which in my family was considered far too racy for a young girl. And on snow days a few times a year, when school was closed, we would go with my dad to help open up the stores so that people could get food, essentials, and gas. We took pride in providing a public service; we were part of the fabric of our town, and we must have looked like it, us kids trailing around after our dad in our hats and mittens, always introducing ourselves to each store clerk. In the snow, my father would attach a ladder on a rope to the back of his car and drive around the neighborhood, and we would pile onto the rungs of the ladder, clinging to it, making it a sled. When he drove just fast enough, it felt like we were riding a magic carpet. The sensation was one of controlled freedom—adventure, but without fear.

Sometimes a boy named Reid would join us for rides on the ladder; he lived on the street that ran parallel to ours, and my father liked to include him, throwing a ball around in the park or kicking a soccer ball together. Reid's father had been paralyzed in an accident years earlier, and now he was in a wheelchair. My father must have felt a kinship with this young man, growing up without a dad who could teach him to play sports.

MY MOTHER'S SIDE OF the family was different—warmer, more emotional. My middle name, Jeannine, was given to me after my maternal grandmother, who was spunky and irreverent. She was my fiercest supporter, always doling out little felt bumblebee stickers as symbols of her affection and pride. She cheered from the stands at all of my games: "Let's go, Amy Jeannine!" There was a note of pride in her voice when she spoke her own name, now mine, out loud. She and my grandfather had a ranch in Oklahoma, four hours' drive from Amarillo, which we called the pig farm, although there were no pigs on it; it was just called that because it was a place to get dirty and have fun.

I would fish with Jeannine on the banks of a little pond, the trees swaying in the breeze, the sun shining on our faces, our butts in the bristly grass, waiting for a catfish to pull down the red-and-white bobber so we could reel in our catch. The minute the fish took the line, my heart would pound— the exhilaration of it, the challenge. My grandmother kept a glass of what looked like watered-down soda next to her. I'd sneak a sip and spit it out—yuck, bourbon!—never learning my lesson.

Jeannine taught me how to drive at the ranch out in Oklahoma when I was twelve years old. I rammed the car into a cattle guard just in time for my father to walk up and witness the driver's side scrape along the metal post. Not knowing how to back up, I kept moving through the gate, hoping the shrill metal crunching sound would just stop. When it finally did, my dad smiled calmly. "Is everyone all right?" he asked, chuckling. We nodded. "Jean, why did you let her drive the car?"

"Well, she had to start somewhere," my grandmother said, laughing.

"Dad, are you mad?" I asked. "I'm so sorry." I didn't want to disappoint him.

"No," he said. He leaned into the open window. "It's only a car. Cars can be fixed. I'm just glad you're all right."

This was my father's rational side: He was always principled, linear in his thinking. If we had to call home in a crisis, we knew that if my mother answered, we should say: "Mom, everyone is alive. Now can I speak to Dad?"

My mother, Julie, had been raised in Enid, Oklahoma,

where she was the May Queen. My grandmother said that my mom was so perfect that as a teenager she gave her a carton of eggs and told her to go throw them at cars. "Just do something naughty," she said, but my mother didn't know how; it wasn't in her nature.

In college, she modeled for the local department store. She was a classic beauty, with thick blond hair like a Barbie doll—volume on top and a curl at the bottom—a straight, angular nose and a smile that conveyed warmth and acceptance. She was wholesome, feminine—an all-American woman. Watching her put on makeup and perfume to go out with my father at night was soothing to me. I was skinny and athletic, with wavy hair that stubbornly refused my efforts to tame it. It was unimaginable to me that I would someday be perceived as pretty or feminine the way my mother was. To me, she was perfect. Both of my parents were: They reminded me of Larry Hagman and Barbara Eden from *I Dream of Jeannie,* and they even looked like them too. Like Major Nelson, my dad was good in a crisis, and like Jeannie, my mother seemed capable of magic.

My parents met at the University of Oklahoma. It was a setup, and my father thought he was going out with my mother's best friend. Instead, my mother came down the staircase at her sorority house. My father took one look at her and thought: *Wow! Not who I expected, but this will do.*

My mother became the quintessential homemaker, tightly French-braiding my hair while watching the *Today* show, the sweet and acidic smell of orange juice from concentrate filling the kitchen, where there was always a glass cloche of homemade cookies, a Bundt cake, or banana pudding made with vanilla wafers and condensed milk. Looking good was important. Our Christmas card was always sent on time, some clever little message over a photo of all of us perfectly dressed; in the process of getting the shot, we all would have pushed, poked, and prodded one another a hundred times, but so long as there was one photo with the four of us smiling, that was all that mattered. Growing up in the South, you understand quickly the ocean that separates appearance and reality, particularly for women. There was an expectation, both ambiently felt and articulated, that women should always look good, even while effortlessly juggling domestic tasks. My grandmother Novie was the only woman I knew who worked, but it set a powerful example because she was entrepreneurial—a dynamo whose presence was felt across West Texas. Never mind that people were edgy around Novie. That was just what happened when you were a boss who happened to be a woman.

As a girl, I absorbed the energy of these adults around me. My father's side was formidable: his mother, this rare woman in a position of power in a conservative, patriarchal world, and my father himself, for whom accomplishments reigned supreme and to whom comparison was not the thief of joy but the only accurate measure of success. On my mother's, there was a different kind of strength: the kind conferred through softness and warmth and generosity and through selfless doing for others, the way my mother took care of us and everyone in town.

From an early age, I was told that I was a natural leader. In some ways, perhaps, it was a birthright: My mother modeled kindness and my father modeled achievement. Leadership, I thought, existed at the crosshairs of these two qualities. There was no higher good than to be good to people. Besides, as I was reminded often, I was very fortunate. I knew to pay it forward. Looking back, I can see that this laid the foundation for the person I would eventually become—a people pleaser, someone who was conditioned to think of others' needs first and who strove to be perceived as a pillar of virtue within the community.

But it was also understood that, along with my siblings, I was an ambassador of the family business. Every time I opened the door to one of the stores and heard the ringing of the overhead bell, I felt that I had entered a place that demanded reverence. The employees knew who I was. I should be respectful and grateful for their service. Others had the luxury of making mistakes. I wanted to make my family proud. By the time I got my driver's license, I had learned to be hypervigilant. "I got a call from store sixty-four," my father said to me one night. "You left your gas cap on the top of the tank when you were filling up this afternoon." The message was clear: People were watching, all the time.

GETTING TO AMARILLO WAS a challenge; you had to fly through Denver or Dallas to get in or get out. From the highway, Amarillo might have looked like little more than a place you would stop for a bathroom break on a long-haul cross-country trip, wedged between truck stops as vast as small cities and the Big Texan steak house, where if you could clear an entire seventy-two-ounce steak with all the trimmings, including dessert, you'd get it for free. But away from the freeway that bisected the town was a real community, a place where people cared about family, God, and sports. And so together they raised their children, prayed, and played.

In a town like Amarillo, athletics were how you got noticed, a ticket out if you wanted one. My father was a natural athlete, and my mother had been a cheerleader. I inherited my father's killer instinct and competitive spirit. My mother made sure the Izod logo always faced the right way on my tennis skirt, and that I shook everyone's hand and looked them in the eye after a match. I played soccer, T-ball, and tennis, did gymnastics, and when I was twelve years old, joined a volleyball team. Around that same time, I began running. I can't recall anyone teaching me how to run, and I don't know that I was good at it. It was just something I always did: I needed to move.

I would throw on a pair of highlighter-yellow wind shorts, an old Lacoste T-shirt, and a pair of Reeboks and leave my bedroom, with its white wicker furniture and matte white Venetian blinds. I'd walk past the bathroom and my sister Lizzie's room, turn left, and head out the front door, past the cherry tree and the brick inlay with the flower bed where red tulips bloomed, a little brighter than the color of the brick, and across five steps. Dividing our property from the neighbor's was a staggered brick wall, one brick wide, the perfect dimension to use as a balance beam or for cartwheels. I would jog down Carter Street, past the Presbyterian church on the corner and along a footpath that cut diagonally through a circular park, on the other side of which was the field where my dad coached my soccer team. At the far end of the park was Navarro Middle School, where I was a student.

I knew the families who lived in every house on our street. There was the orange brick house that belonged to the man who owned a Burger King franchise in town. There was the house where a kind, elderly man with a walker always bought Girl Scout cookies from me. My brother Jeff's best friend lived in the house on the corner. Mary Lou Davidson, who was the most gracious woman in town and who always had homemade ice cream on hand, lived right across the street; she had a circular driveway, and she didn't mind if we used it as the neighborhood racetrack, maybe because her children were grown and she lived alone. The family in the house next to us on the left would always generously sponsor me when I was asking for pledges for Jump Rope for Heart, an annual school fundraiser.

We were instructed by our teachers that if people invited us in while we were going door to door, we should politely tell them that we preferred to stay outside. This would keep us safe. This was important to me, growing up, as it was to us all. When I ran down my street, I would look at each of the doors as I passed by, knowing that the people inside were familiar to me; if a windowless white van were to approach in an attempt to kidnap me, as seemed to happen often to little girls I heard about on the five o'clock news, I could run inside and ask anyone in these homes for help. Our neighbors were friendly. Trustworthy. Good.

I would run around the perimeter of the park, along the walkway that took me by the school, around the tennis courts, the whole circle in a loop. But I never set foot on the grass that was technically school grounds—I'd only run around it, then back to my house. It was like I wanted to pretend the school wasn't there.

It wasn't as if I were unhappy at school; I was popular and well-liked, a star athlete, and always told I set a good example for the rest of the class. My volleyball coach, Coach Taylor, who was young and peppy and always wore her hair in a ponytail, would often say to the team, "Everyone, look at Amy," when she was trying to get the other girls to participate in a drill or execute a pass in a certain way. The only thing holding me back was my gender, since I knew that in the larger game of life, girls rarely won.

In the spring, when election season came around, I decided to run for president of the student council. I was sure that I would lose, but at least it would make a statement that I had run at all. "Everyone knows a boy will win," I told my best friend Rachel. "Girls usually run for secretary so they can take the notes."

"You really don't think you can win?" Rachel asked, clicking her retainer up and down in her mouth. In the second grade, she had knocked one of her front teeth out on the playground, and the whole class spent an hour sifting through the pebbles like archaeologists in the field, trying to find the missing tooth, to no avail. Now she wore a flipper, which she would sometimes remove as a party trick to spook unsuspecting boys.

"No chance," I said.

I was right: A boy named Bradley Jones won instead. I liked Bradley—in fact, I had a crush on him—but there was no doubt in my mind I would have done a better job.

After I lost the election, one of my favorite teachers in the school, Mr. Mason, stopped me in the hallway. "We all know you're the real leader of this school," he said. I pulled my shoulders back, standing up straighter. These words of praise put a new spring in my step. I felt like he was seeing me for who I really was. Now I was a part of the group. He had confirmed what I believed myself to be, the same thing my parents expected me to be. All I had to do was continue living up to that title. *The real leader of this school.*

So I arrived at practice early. I paid attention at all times, even when other kids were distracted. I stayed late at school, so late that the only people left in the building were

Coach Taylor and Mr. Mason; I remember watching him pull out of the faculty parking lot, his elbow on the sill of the rolled-down car window, waving goodbye as I stood on the curb. That I was staying later than even the teachers was a testament to my commitment. I even organized the volleyball team to purchase a gift for Coach Taylor—a James Avery ring with a cross on it, which we pooled our money to buy. When we presented it to her, she was moved to tears.

Doing nice things for others made me feel good about myself; it was something my parents had modeled. There was a girl in my grade named Claudia who had blue eyes and blunt-cut bangs; I understood that her home life was turbulent. A few weeks before cotillion, I learned that Claudia didn't have a dress to wear. "I'll lend you a dress," I said. "I have two options—a floral one and a pink one. Which do you want?" The joy I felt to be able to offer Claudia that dress was boundless. The thought of her feeling special wearing it made me feel special.

When I saw Claudia in the floral dress with puffy sleeves the night of the dance, I smiled at her and flashed her a thumbs-up. She looked beautiful. But when she looked back at me, her eyes were clouded, vulnerable, as if she were afraid I might reveal her secret. I wanted to tell her that I would never tell anyone that the dress she was wearing wasn't her own; doing that would undermine how good it felt to lend it to her. I knew how to keep a secret.

THERE WAS ONE MEMORY that replayed on a loop in my mind for years. On the day we graduated from eighth grade, Coach Taylor stood to give the highest student award of the year, which was for leadership—not just scholastic achievement but also kindness. The winner would have their photo framed on the wall in the main hallway of the school for years to come. As she spoke, touting the accomplishments of a student who was hardworking, dedicated, and inspiring to her peers, her voice cracked and she began to cry.

Then she looked at me. I heard my name, but I couldn't move.

"Amy, it's you," the friend sitting next to me said. "You have to go up there."

I stood up, looked around, and made my way to the stage. Time seemed to move in slow motion. I felt both overwhelmed and numb. Up there, looking out at the crowd, I saw my parents looking back at me, clapping. Time stopped. Tears streamed down my father's face. I had never seen him cry before.

Why do I remember this so clearly? It wasn't about the award. The image of my parents' pride, their joy in me, stayed so vivid in my mind because it was the moment I knew that I was the living fulfillment of their dreams. I was to exemplify their finest qualities. I was supposed to be the brightest—perfect.

Memory is a sieve that catches only the most important moments. The insignificant details of daily life don't stick; instead, they flow through the sieve. Then there are experiences that are unusual, set apart from the everyday, that carry an emotional charge. These we often hold on to, turning them over and over. As I do with this image. The roar of the applause, the tears in my father's eyes, and me standing onstage. Everyone was looking at me. I should have been so happy. But instead, I felt utterly alone. It was as if the girl they were looking at wasn't me at all.

. . .

I UNDERSTOOD THAT, AS much as I wanted to lead, there would be limits to my power because I was a girl. My father told me that if I could drive a stick-shift car and learn to ski, I would always have a date. Driving stick was particularly important, he said, because I should be able to drive myself home if my date had too much to drink. So he taught me how to drive on the sandy roads of the Palo Duro Canyon near the dam, where all the water would dry up if there hadn't been any rain. He was patient with me as I spun my tires out in the sand. "Shift," he would say. "Now shift again." I followed his direction. "Now let's go try it on the hill again." I wasn't just learning how to drive. I was learning how to be self-sufficient, and in being self-sufficient, I would be safe.

Amarillo was right in the middle of Tornado Alley; the threat of storms was omnipresent. We had tornado drills at school where the alarm would sound, a trilling bell that shrieked and shrieked. We would shut all the doors and go out into the hallways, facing the lockers. The girls would crouch down on the ground, and the boys would crouch over them with their elbows pressed against the lockers. This didn't bother me at the time. I thought it was nice that girls were to be protected, even if there was a secondary, tacit message: We were not strong enough on our own.

I didn't think about any of this too much: I knew that I was strong. My mother used to joke that I could have run the CIA as a child. "You always thought you were better than us," my sister, Lizzie, said once. Early on, Lizzie had struggled to find her footing in school; when I came home, I'd always find my mother in Lizzie's bedroom, helping her with her homework. Late into the night, I could hear them work-ing together side by side, writing an essay or studying for a spelling test. I didn't like the idea of asking for help, although I was jealous of the time they spent together.

When Lizzie accused me of thinking I was better than her, of course, I denied it. But at some level, Lizzie was right. I worked harder than most of my peers. I pushed myself more. Wasn't that what it meant to be better? The way pres-sure makes a diamond, I thought that striving for exception-alism, no matter how burdensome it felt at times, was a virtue. It was my superpower.

But it weighed on me. Everything had to be perfect. Not just at home but everywhere. Even when I went away to summer camp, my clothes had to be meticulously folded in my trunk, personal items tucked neatly away in my Jon Hart bag, the one with my name on it. My bedspread had to be thin enough that you could see the crease where it lined up with the mattress, a show of perfect symmetry. If other kids didn't pick up their shoes during camp inspection, I felt a surge of nerves. While everyone else was watching movies at the outdoor amphitheater, I would run laps around the track, making good use of my time. At night, I would lie in bed stressing about what medals I would take home. Would I win the canoe race? Would that be enough? Looking back, I can see that I was ruled by fear. Yet this made no sense: What was there to be afraid of?

The mere thought of misbehaving ratcheted up my anxi-ety. In high school, kids would get drunk and hook up on one particular block in my neighborhood; those of us on the volleyball team weren't allowed to be seen getting out of a car there or even driving by the spot. When I was a sophomore, my other best friend, Courtney—who was confident, whip-smart, and could hold a pencil in her curled bangs—got caught merely hanging out on that street, and she had to run three miles each morning before school as punishment. There was no way I would ever do something so reckless.

Other kids seemed to have an easygoing approach to life that was incomprehensible to me. Even Hikari, the fastidiously polite Japanese exchange student who spent a year living with Courtney's family, seemed to be having more fun than I was: During an actual tornado warning, sirens blaring through the neighborhood, Courtney found dozens of crushed beer cans under his bed in her basement. He'd come to America for a cultural experience, and he was certainly having one. Why couldn't I, in my own hometown?

It wasn't that I was serious all the time. Rachel and I took woodshop solely so we could hang out with the cute boys. At sleepovers, Courtney and I would prank-call the neighbors. "Is your refrigerator running?" she'd ask. "*Then you better go catch it!*" she'd shriek as we howled with laughter. The three of us would pick up burritos at Taco Villa, the local Mexican fast-food restaurant, where you'd have to lean halfway out the car window to scream your order into the speaker, spelling out B-E-A-N or B-E-E-F, since they sounded the same. The ridiculousness of the drive-through was half the fun.

But as I grew older, I was too dogged to do something as reckless as going out drinking with kids my own age. "Blame it on me," my dad would say when I worried about saying no to an invitation to go drinking out at the lake. "Use me as the scapegoat." So I'd tell my friends that my parents were really strict. It was true, at least of my father, who would wait by the front door, arms crossed, at curfew so I'd see his disapproval if I was even a minute late; he was trying to keep me safe. But the truth was, I was the real taskmaster. I knew that what I was rejecting when I didn't go out was the unpredictability of not knowing what might happen. In high school, I had this sense that, increasingly, there were things that could get us into trouble, particularly involving drinking or sex. I never wanted anyone to see me with my defenses down. I had to stay in control and be a good girl—and a leader.

Yet in committing to that, I became rigid. That looseness, that spontaneity that I'd felt as a little girl, jumping on my banana-seat bike or doing cartwheels on the soccer field— somewhere along the way, I'd lost it. It had been supplanted by teenage neurosis and an insidious need for control, but I wasn't sure how or when that had happened. It was like I'd blinked and my childhood freedom had vanished.

Maybe that was just what growing up felt like—to lose that innocence and disinhibition, to replace them with an adult-minded sense of responsibility. *Just work three times harder than everyone else,* I would say to myself when I got out of bed in the morning. There was always another hoop to jump through, always another carrot dangling. I never stopped to ask myself why. I thought that was just how life worked: a series of challenges to be met and boxes to be checked. When I would play tennis against my father, he'd tell me he'd buy me a new tennis outfit if I could beat him. Then he started promising me a red sports car if I didn't go on a date until I was sixteen. Every time a zippy red convertible drove by the house, he would look over at me. "There it is," he'd say half jokingly. "Only a few years away."

On my sixteenth birthday, he brought me to a repo car lot owned by a family friend, where there were perhaps fifty cars. Then he pulled a set of keys from his pocket, jangling them in his hand.

"These are the keys to your car," he said, smiling. "You get three guesses as to which one I picked out for you. If you don't get it right, we'll come back another day." He seemed pleased with his game. I looked around the lot, scanning the aisles of cars—late-model or rusted, flashy or practical. My eye landed on a blue, two-door Chevy Blazer. I knew instantly that was the car he'd picked out for me; I could read him like a book. It was safe and modest.

But what if he'd actually delivered on the red sports car? Hope springs eternal.

I pointed to a fire-engine-red Mazda Miata. "That one," I said.

"Go and try it," he said. So I walked over to the car and tried the key in the ignition. It wouldn't budge. I looked back at him. He smiled, watching me.

I pointed to a sleek coupe. He shrugged his shoulders as if to say: *Maybe.* I walked over to it and turned the key again. No luck.

Then I went to the Blazer. I slid the key into the ignition, turned it, and felt the car start. I looked back at my father. He was grinning. Of course, it was generous; my father was always generous. And even though I hadn't gone on any dates, earning the red sports car he'd promised, we'd both always known that had been a joke. I was grateful for the Blazer. Still, the gift wasn't freely given. Even this was presented as a kind of ceremonial challenge—a game I had to win.

I understood that having my own car was a big deal and an important rite of passage. Behind the wheel, staring out at the long, flat landscape, with Garth Brooks blaring on the radio and the dash slick with Armor All, Texas sun shining through the windshield, I felt a new sense of freedom. But this freedom wasn't what I'd felt as a little girl on my banana-seat bike; the definition had changed. Back then, freedom was a kind of abandon—wild, reckless, unselfconscious. Now I felt free when I could control every detail, from the temperature to the song on the stereo to where I would go next.

BY MY SENIOR YEAR of high school, I was the school president, captain of the volleyball team, and in the top 2 percent of my class. I was nominated to the homecoming court, where I hoped—maybe even expected—that I would be crowned queen. No one knew what qualified you for the title. Was it beauty? Was it behavior? The opacity only made it more important to me—a game with no discernible rules that I still had to figure out how to win.

I was paraded onto the football field in a long, fitted black halter dress with a fake diamond choker around the neck. I wore high heels, which I'd worn only a handful of times before and which I knew would be ruined as they sank into the sod—a necessary sacrifice for the pageantry of the day. I walked to the center of the field to pose next to a football player I didn't know very well in front of the thousands of people in the crowd. Reserve officers in military uniforms with raised swords clustered on either side of us, adding to the sense of theater.

A marching band played, loud and jangly, and the sun was hot and direct. I smiled and waved, as was my responsibility. I looked up into the stands, understanding that I was an object. The announcer's voice crackled through the speakers, muffled by the howl of the West Texas winds.

Then they called not my name but someone else's. A girl named Jane, who was the head cheerleader and now homecoming queen. I bit the sides of my mouth and smiled on.

The feeling was one of sudden death. This was a popularity contest, and I had lost. There was no Mr. Mason to tell me that I was the real leader of this school. I was being put out to pasture. I went home and wept. Then I fixed my makeup and went to the homecoming dance.

It wasn't just that I felt that I had fallen short, although I did. This was something deeper than that. I felt exposed and ashamed. Losing the homecoming queen title confirmed some private, ugly unworthiness that I had been working so hard to keep anyone from seeing. Why hadn't I won? I had tried so hard to be perfect.

The past is full of paradoxes. I knew that I was loved by my parents. Even my name, Amy, meant *beloved*. I was reminded of it every time I looked at the turquoise bag from Joan Altman's, the Jon Hart bag with my name on it. I loved my family and I loved my friends. My connections were deep and real.

But at some point I had come to believe that I was loved not for any inherent worth but because of all my accomplishments. With each new accomplishment came more praise; that praise, I thought, *was* love. Yet I burned through the praise so quickly: There was never enough to sustain me. I was constantly looking for my next hit of validation. I needed people to affirm that what I was working so hard for was worth it, that I was separate from the crowd.

So I thought it made sense that when I searched my

memory, so much of what I saw was myself, alone. What remained in the sieve was solitude, isolation. I was always running, my bleach-white sneakers pounding the old foot-path through that park down the street from my house. I had memories of standing on the curb in the parking lot outside school, or the way the afternoon light sliced through the hall-way outside the history room as I walked down it, alone, hav-ing stayed late again.

Maybe that wasn't surprising. Perfection is a lonely pur-suit.

FROM THE OUTSIDE, MY life looked perfect. On some level, I must have believed that it was. But I see now that there are parts of the story that I was missing. I realize that there are things I believed because they were convenient, and I had been brought up to think that's what made them good. It's nice when things are packaged, and easy, and clean, isn't it? The athlete, the good girl, the natural leader. Convenience. Perfection.

Nothing in life is free.

Everything has a cost.

2. DANGER

I ran on the campus at the University of Virginia, up and down verdant hills, the landscape lush and clotted with yellow-leaved gingkoes and dogwoods in full bloom. There were so many trees it was almost claustrophobic. The dry expanse of the Panhandle felt a million miles away. One day, my volleyball coach pulled me aside with a furrowed brow. I felt intuitively that she didn't like me, although I didn't know why. "I've seen how much you run," she said. "It's ruining your vertical jump." She told me to stop running more than three miles a day. I didn't want to get in trouble, but I needed to get faster and stronger if I wanted to stay competitive, and I didn't trust her judgment. So I started taking routes where I knew she wouldn't see me, running in secret through the campus.

I had been admitted to UVA on a volleyball scholarship, and I knew my parents were proud of me for getting into a good school, even if my father seemed to have reservations about my going so far away. My parents had hoped that I would stay closer to home—maybe go to their alma mater—but I wanted to expand my horizons. Most of my classmates were staying in the state; leaving was the exception, not the rule. As I was packing up, my father gave me a dozen yellow roses. "Don't forget about Texas," he said. I would never forget about Texas—it was my home. But the world beyond was shiny, and I was eager to explore it.

I loved everything about college. The campus was historic and grand, and the students were different from the kids I'd grown up with in Amarillo. They seemed scholarly and civic-minded, open and progressive. I wanted to study English; maybe, I thought, I would become a journalist, like Diane Sawyer or Katie Couric—strong women I'd grown up watching, whom I knew to be truth tellers in the face of injustice or hypocrisy. As a student athlete, I learned to multitask. There was never enough time to organize my thoughts before I wrote my papers; I bullet-pointed assignments in my head while I was doing other things. The volleyball team swam for conditioning several times a week, and it was there, in the water, in the meditative monotony of crossing back and forth in the pool, that I could think clearly, writing in my head. After climbing out, I'd rush back to my dorm room, hair still dripping wet, to clack out the words on my laptop. The computer was heavy and prone to overheating; often while I wrote on long bus trips to conference games, it would get so hot that I'd have to stack a pillow and several books on my lap to keep it from burning my legs.

My first semester in college, I took a class from a beloved psychology professor named Raymond Bice; everyone called his class "Bice Psych," and the enrollment was huge, a class of hundreds. One day, he was teaching a unit on memory. "I'm going to show you something today that you will never forget," he said. "And I know you'll never forget it, because memory is specific. You remember a moment. A thing. A visual. An object."

He held up a teddy bear. It was so big he had trouble lifting it over his head. "I can guarantee you one thing when you think of this class," he said from behind the stuffed animal. "You may have forgotten everything else, but you will always remember this." He was right. The image of that giant stuffed bear has stayed with me for the rest of my life, something I couldn't forget if I tried.

AFTER MY FIRST YEAR at college, I spent the summer in Austin. I ran there too, around the lake, stopping to look at the canopy of bats chirping under the bridge, or on the treadmill when it was too hot to be outside. I had landed an internship at the capitol working for Amarillo's representative in the Texas Senate, but they were out of session, so there was nothing to do. I wore pantyhose and skirts to the capitol every day, as was expected of women there, and carried buckets of ice to the office of anyone who called for it, since the building wasn't air-conditioned. I gained no real work experience, but that was never the point; it was about being able to put on my résumé that I had worked there.

A friend of my mother's set me up on a date with a former college football star. He drove a white Blazer and wore a gold chain around his neck, which wasn't my type, but he was good-looking, and I wanted him to like me. We went out many times, but he never kissed me. "I don't think I should," he said once.

"Why not?" I asked. I felt ashamed. I wondered if there was something wrong with me.

"Because I'm an all-or-nothing kind of guy," he said. "If you're not going to have sex with me, then I shouldn't kiss you. I can't stop myself." I couldn't argue with his reasoning, especially considering there was no chance that I would have sex with him.

Sex was utterly foreign to me. I had been taught what my body parts were but not how they worked or how to use them. I can still recall the specific humiliation of having to get my parents' permission when we took sex ed in the fifth grade; I kept the permission slip in my backpack until the day it was due, getting it signed at the last minute. Even with my closest friends, Rachel and Courtney, we never talked about sex. Our romantic fantasies were of being courted by boys, which had less to do with the levers of our own desire than it did with finding the answer to the omnipresent question: *Do you think he likes me?* This was important: We had to wait to see if boys were going to choose us. We knew never to pursue someone first; it was better to be pursued. If anyone in my high school was having sex, I was naïve to it; my friends and I were still conditioned, as proper southern girls, not to talk about it, even with one another.

As for my parents, they were less than forthcoming about what went on between adults. In my house growing up, I wasn't allowed to call a boy—he would have to call me first. As I got out of the car with my father when I was not yet a teen, on my way to a tennis lesson, he said: "Your mother was a virgin when I married her, and I expect you to be the same." I froze, uncomfortable at the mere mention of virginity. I couldn't bear to look back to see the expression on his face.

"Uh-huh," I said. "Got it." As quickly as I could, I slung my racket bag over my shoulder and closed the door firmly behind me.

It was bred into you, between school, church, and southern morality, that a woman was meant to look pretty, take care of the kids, and somehow maintain the appearance of chastity while doing it. Boys were wolves pursuing their prey; girls should protect their purity until it was torn from them by the force of male lust, not their own desire or agency. My mother was always skittish about people approaching her from behind; it wasn't until I was a teenager that my dad told me the story of how, when my mom was a high school senior, the milkman surprised her in the kitchen, throwing her to the floor in an attempted assault. She screamed and fought him off. "So it's not that I don't trust *you*," my father would say. "It's the guys I don't trust."

In my experience, my father was right to mistrust the boys. My high school boyfriend always seemed to want more from me than I was comfortable giving. Once, at a party, he led me into a bathroom so we could make out. I could feel that, like any hormonal teenage boy, he wanted as much as I was willing to give, but I felt claustrophobic and afraid. I flung the door open and bolted away from him, back to the safety of my friends.

I never slept with him. My culture had taught me that my virginity was sacred—the ultimate prize. It was my responsibility to protect and mine alone.

The principles of achievement I applied to academics and athletics also applied to sex. My understanding of romance existed at the intersection of the patriarchy that raised me and my father's paradigm of accomplishments, where the best was expected and everything became a game that could be won through hard work and determination. To prove my merit, I needed to be chosen by a man—someone special, someone powerful. To be wanted would confirm my value. I had my own desires—I knew that I liked guys who were tall, confident, and funny—but those were secondary concerns. What really mattered was that I cultivate the credentials that would make someone like me, that I become salable to the world of men who would determine my worth. Hopefully someone would find me more valuable than I'd been that day on the football field when I'd lost the homecoming crown.

That summer in Austin, I lived in a big shared house near the University of Texas with several other girls. I was bunking with a girl named Sarah, who was from Dallas; she was a year older than I was and a fellow visiting student. We had been assigned a sparsely furnished room with two twin beds, since we were both only there for the summer. One night I came home after having been out with friends. When I arrived back at the house and went upstairs to my bedroom, Sarah was still out. It was late, but I was hungry, so I went downstairs to rummage around in the kitchen for a snack.

I fished around in the pantry until I found some graham crackers. I ate them idly, looking out the sliding glass door into the backyard. Suddenly, I couldn't shake the feeling that someone was watching me. I couldn't see anyone out the door, but I felt it—an eerie, instinctual knowing. I realized that I was wearing only a T-shirt and my underwear, and I felt stupid and irresponsible for being half dressed where someone might see me, for allowing myself to be this exposed and vulnerable. I wanted to check that the door was locked but knew that none of us carried a key, so that was the only entry for the other girls to come home later in the night. Instead, carefully, I left the kitchen, went upstairs, and got into bed, pulling the covers over my head. Surely, I convinced myself, it was all in my head. Eventually, fear still tight in my body, I fell asleep.

In the night, I awakened to the sound of screaming. It was as high-pitched and shrill as a tornado drill. I looked out to see that the bedroom door was wide open. Then I looked over and saw that Sarah's bed was empty. I bolted up. "What's happening?" I screamed. I heard doors slamming, then girls' voices yelling, overlapping, a panicked choir.

"Stay in your room! Stay in your room!"

I slammed the door and slid down onto the floor. My whole body shook.

After coming home, Sarah had gone downstairs to get a glass of water, and she'd run into an intruder with a pair of pantyhose over his head. They tussled on the hardwood floor, and he then fled, leaving the pantyhose stuck to the back fence. Eventually the police caught him, a serial rapist who assaulted fourteen women over the course of two years in Austin, holding them down with knives.

Traumatized and covered in bruises, Sarah ended up going home to Dallas for the rest of the summer. The other girls and I never processed our feelings about the incident. We barely spoke about it to one another, nor did I ever unpack what had happened with Sarah when I saw her at a wedding years later. Even though we had all been there, the experience was so violating that it was easier to pretend it had never happened. Instead, we brought a guard dog from the home of one of the other girls—a Labrador who snoozed by the front door all day and night as we stepped over him to leave the house.

With sex, as I understood it, there was a terrible push and pull. Men wished to take something from you—your purity, your chastity, your goodness—and would endeavor to do so, by force if necessary. As a woman it was your duty to defend it. If you failed, you would only have yourself to blame. I never slept in only a T-shirt and underwear again.

STUDYING ABROAD IN EUROPE the summer after my sophomore year, I ran a six-mile loop every day through a park in Valencia. My host family gossiped about me in Spanish: "All she does is run," they said, which made me sad. I'd imagined connecting with their three daughters, but all they seemed to want to do was watch soap operas on the couch night after night; they had no interest in me.

Toward the end of the trip, I traveled to Ibiza with a group of girls, catching a cheap ride on an overnight barge. We went out to a club that was filled with foam, which was like walking around an enormous empty bathtub, with women carrying trays of Jell-O shots. Clubgoers had live snakes wrapped around their necks and neon bracelets on their wrists. I surveyed the room like an anthropologist; everyone was dripping in suds and sex, but I was guarded.

In the morning, we took a bus across the island. Most of the group hadn't slept, and the vehicle was hot and badly air-

conditioned. When we got out, blinking at the harsh sunlight, we made our way in the direction of a beach that was
known to be stunning. "It's a bit of a hike to get to this spot,"
one of the girls said, "but once you get there, it's so special."

As we cleared the top of a hill, we descended onto the
most pristine beach I'd ever seen, vast and golden. It was a
windless morning, the water flat and warm and clear. The
women were topless, their skin reddened from the sun, their
breasts exposed. Their bodies were sultry; just by virtue of
being Spanish, they seemed more sensuous than us pale,
repressed Americans. I felt a pinch of anxiety: Were we all
going to go topless, too? But it was the culturally appropriate
thing, and so we stripped off our bathing suit tops and lay on
the sand, reveling in the sun, free. From a thatched shack set
back from the beach, I ate the freshest salad I'd ever tasted,
made with mango, corn, and avocado; it was sweet and salty.

Later in the day, I went out swimming by myself. I turned
away from the group, tilting my face toward the sun, looking
out to the horizon. I was truly happy. I felt like the most essential version of myself: free in my body, the way I'd been as
a little girl doing cartwheels, unburdened by expectations. It
was a day that would be etched in my memory forever. I dove
into the crystalline water, then returned to the surface, pressing my hair back out of my face and wiping the salt from my
eyes.

Then I turned back to the shore. I saw now that there was
a group of boys walking along the water's edge, kicking at
the sand with their bare feet as they carried their sneakers in
their hands. Their close-cropped haircuts, their oversize
backpacks, and the way they traveled in a pack, loudly chat-
tering, told me instantly that they were American.

Reflexively, at the sight of them, I put my hands across my bare breasts. It wasn't something I thought about. It was just something that I knew to do, an animal instinct.

ON ANOTHER SUMMER BREAK, I spent six weeks studying in London. It was my first time in Britain, and I was living in a dormitory in Regent's Park surrounded by rose gardens that were supposedly beloved by Princess Diana, which struck me as terribly romantic. I ran through the park in the summer heat on pathways cut between the rosebushes—their deep reds, cheerful yellows, and creamy whites. I memorized the names of the roses as I ran, looking down at their plaques: *Lady of Shalott. Tickled pink. Southern belle.*

After I'd been there a few days, my father called. "Listen," he said. "I've got something fun for you to do while you're over there." His tone suggested Diana herself might be requesting an audience with me. My father had never been to London, not because he didn't like to travel or couldn't afford it; he just liked spending time on the ranch or going to places that were accessible by car.

"What is it?" I asked.

"Remember that group of guys from Austin I go hunting with once a year?"

"Yes, of course," I said.

"Well, I ran into one of them, and he mentioned that his son James is in London working for a bank this summer. Can I connect the two of you?"

"Yeah, that sounds great. Thanks, Dad," I said.

The next week, James called to ask if I wanted to go see a Premier League game with him. I was excited to experience a soccer match on its home turf. But more than that, I could tell it gratified my father to know his connections could grant me an opportunity all the way on the other side of the Atlantic.

James was good-looking and cocky, which reminded me of the men back home in Texas. Going to a football match on a Saturday in London felt like making a pilgrimage to a sacred site, thousands of spectators gathering to watch eleven little men kick a black-and-white ball across an expanse of field. The real show was in the stands, the red-faced fans chanting and praying to the soccer gods. After the match, James leaned in close to me.

"So, we're two Texans in England—what are you doing after this?" he said. "Can I take you to dinner?"

I nodded. I was in a foreign country, which felt exotic, and my father already approved of James's family. This was exactly the type of man to whom I should say yes.

We went to an Italian restaurant, where we drank a bottle of red wine. I had just turned twenty-one and didn't have much experience drinking beyond strawberry wine coolers, cheap frat-party beer, and the occasional margarita. But it felt glamorous and sophisticated to be swirling wine in my glass with my last-minute date. He'd gone to an Ivy League school; I told him how I'd told all my friends I was going to college on the East Coast when I got into the University of Virginia, not realizing just how southern it actually was. But to a girl from West Texas, Charlottesville was still a long way from home.

After dinner, we walked a short distance back to the flat James had rented, which was dated, outfitted in institutional brown and green. More wine flowed as we talked until late in the evening. When he leaned in to kiss me, I kissed him back. Then I looked at my watch. It was past 1:00 A.M. How was I going to extract myself gracefully? I realized that I was far from my dorm, and I was drunk. Taking the tube that late at night was dangerous; how would I find my way? I knew that black cabs were expensive.

"You're welcome to stay here with me," James said, like a true southern gentleman. "But don't feel any pressure." I felt safe with him. He was from back home. I would stay.

Wine-drunk, hands all over each other, we made our way toward the bedroom. "Where is your favorite place you've had sex?" James asked as we passed through the doorway. The question caught me off guard. I fumbled for an answer, stammering.

"In a hot tub," I said finally. I knew it sounded stupid as soon as I'd said it, but I hoped he would move on and not press the matter further.

We tumbled into bed. Everything felt hazy. The sheets billowed around us. Then I felt my senses returning to me as I realized what was happening.

"No," I said. "James, no. No. No. No." The room was spinning. I was frozen, immobile. I felt as if I were in a vacuum. I floated somewhere above my body, feeling sorry for the girl in that bed. It was the exact same feeling I'd had in my middle school auditorium when my name was called all those years earlier, feeling exposed and ashamed, disconnected somehow, as though it were happening to someone else—some other girl. That girl should have paid for the black cab. She should have asked for a blanket and slept on the couch. She should have known this was coming. She should never have had that last glass of wine. She should never have walked back to his flat in the first place. *What would her father say?*

I was aware, vaguely, of what was happening; the green sheets crumpled around us, but I felt nothing until he stopped moving. Then I began to cry.

"James," I cried, "I said no." I turned away from him so he wouldn't see my tears and lay on my side. There was stillness between us. The sheets no longer moved like waves. The first sign of gray summer light peeked in through the blinds.

"Why are you crying?" he said.

"That was my first time," I said.

"Oh," he said. He sighed. "If I had known it was your first time, I never would have done that." I was silent. "You told me your favorite place to have sex was in a hot tub. I did wonder how that was even possible." Wordlessly, I rolled out of the bed, gathered my clothes, and tumbled from his flat into the dawn.

That morning, back at my dorm, I lay in my bunk bed curled up in a ball until there was a knock on my door. "Amy, phone's for you," a girl in the hall said. "Someone named James."

I sprang out of bed, knowing he was going to make everything right. He had to; it was the only logical solution. I anticipated his somber tone and heartfelt apology. This was the moment, I thought, where he would say how much he realized that he liked me and that he wanted to make it up to me, to take me on a second date and win me over. He was southern, smart, and felt familiar. I couldn't wait to tell my dad that we were dating now. *You'll never guess who I'm dating. Yes, James! We've had the most divine few months. I was so excited to tell you!*

It was imperative that I find some way to shift the narrative to make it tolerable—to transform James into a white knight in my mind.

I twisted the phone cord around my wrist nervously as he spoke. "Amy, hi—how are you?" he said. "I wanted to tell you that, um, I didn't use anything."

"You didn't use anything?" I said. I didn't know what he meant.

"I'm working around the clock while I'm here, so it's just not something I can deal with," he said. Something *he* could deal with? I was still confused.

"You need to get it taken care of, all right?" he said finally. "Just in case." Then I understood.

I nodded silently. The receiver of the phone felt heavy in my hand. Somehow the call was worse than what he had done the night before. But as usual, I would do what was asked of me. It would never have occurred to me that I had a choice.

My roommate took me to a clinic, where I got the morning-after pill. I told the nurse that my boyfriend was in London for the summer working at a bank. I felt no self-pity, only shame. I had given up everything I had been told was important in life for a man who thought so little of me. How could I have allowed that to happen, and all so fast?

A few days later, James called me again and invited me to dinner. I accepted the invitation. Even if he was only pursuing me out of guilt, his interest in me made me feel less used. I had sex with him several more times over the course of the summer. I thought that doing so would make him want me more. By sleeping with him, I could become pleasing to him and neutralize the ugliness of what he'd done to me. But it didn't seem to work. "Why don't you ever move when we have sex?" he asked me once. It had never occurred to me that I should be moving, or feeling any sensation at all. When we had sex, I left my body.

One night when we were together, I drank too much on purpose because I knew what I wanted to say and that I wouldn't have the courage to say it sober. "If my dad knew what you did to me," I said, "he would kill you." I can't remember the look on James's face or what he said in reply, only how it felt to say those words out loud—to release the rage within, to reveal the pain I felt over what had been taken from me.

THE SPRING BEFORE I graduated from college, I went to New York to look for a job. *Sex and the City* was on the air at the time, and I watched it avidly; the opening credits, with that jaunty music and the shot of Carrie getting splashed as the bus passes her by, captivated me. There was a fairy tale to be experienced in New York, I thought. Like so many other young women, I was drawn magnetically to what seemed like a glamorous, exciting fantasy of a big, complicated life in the greatest city in the world.

I stayed with a friend who had grown up in the city. Upon arriving at her apartment, she pulled me into the back bedroom, where she was giggling on the bed with another friend, talking about a party we'd all been invited to that evening. "I ordered pizza," she said. "I'm just waiting for it to get here." She winked at me.

"Oh, great," I said. "I'm starving."

When the doorbell rang, the two girls ran to the front door to greet the pizza delivery guy, enthusiastic as if it were their last meal. Then they ferried the pizza back to the bed-room. I wondered why they weren't taking it to the kitchen, but no matter—I was hungry. *My first slice of New York pizza!* I could almost taste it.

When they opened the box, I saw that instead of a pizza, inside there was a small bag of rolled joints. I had never smoked pot before, and I was terrified of it—to say nothing of my irritation that it wasn't pizza—so I just stood anxiously in the corner of the room and watched while the other girls lifted the window to get high. Drugs were illegal. What if we got arrested? Yet this was the New York life I'd wanted: adult, different from Amarillo, with a hint of danger.

I found a job selling reprints of articles for a media company and moved into an apartment in the West Village with Rachel and three other college friends. The five of us lived in a one-bedroom that had been converted into a space for five by adding temporary walls. The day that I arrived in the city, the streets were filled with men in costumes, carrying brightly colored flags and coated in glitter. "Is this what New York is like on the weekends?" I asked one of my new room-mates, bewildered.

She laughed. "It's the Pride parade," she said, shaking her head. "Think of it as your welcome party."

There was so much from which I had been perfectly in-sulated by the culture of a small town—so much that was new in a big city, that required me to pay attention. I moved to New York to have a relationship with the city, and the en-ergy of it felt like a balm to my nervous system: Just like me, the city was constantly in motion. It was difficult enough to navigate the subway system, to learn how to order coffee at a deli in less than two seconds, and to figure out all three airports when you wanted to leave. LaGuardia was closest, which meant the lowest cab fare; on a good day, you could land in Newark, which baffled me since it was in another state entirely; but for some reason, all the best-timed flights were out of JFK. I had always found it irksome that there were so few direct flights from Amarillo to anywhere else in the country. To be in New York, where three airports could take you directly to anywhere in the world, felt like a form of freedom—a portal to endless possibilities.

The company I worked for published, among other titles, *Ms.* magazine. My office was in a closet, but it was still thrilling to feel like I was a part of something, especially when Gloria Steinem walked down the hallway. I would flatten myself against the wall, too intimidated to even breathe in her direction; she was a feminist icon, and I revered her. I joined a book club with other young professional women who were new to the city, went to alumni events, and spent Sundays wandering through museums or reading fashion magazines in bed. Occasionally I went to church with southern girlfriends. Or I would get a bagel and cream cheese and walk around the flea market in Chelsea, looking for things: an end table that could be repainted for our apartment or an old vase that could be converted into a lamp. I was thrifty, and I had loved hunting for treasure since I was a little girl, scouring antiques stores for majolica plates with my mom and grandmother.

Coming from a place that was so flat, the verticality of New York City boggled my mind; I often felt like a tourist in my own city. I had goals: to ascend the ranks of publishing; to find the best place in the city to have brunch; to stop randomly getting pink eye, as happened several times my first year in New York, most likely from not washing my hands after riding the subway.

But mostly I was just trying to stay in motion. I kept running. Some nights I ran along the West Side Highway. One night a man flashed me. His eyes were shrouded by a hood. I bolted off the running path, making my way through the Meatpacking District back to my apartment. It was before the neighborhood had been gentrified, so there were still carcasses hanging from hooks, blood running in the cobblestone streets. It would never have occurred to me to take a taxi; I was young, on a tight budget, and doing things for myself, no matter how irresponsibly.

My only moments of pause were in yoga classes. The room was always so hot that it was nearly intolerable, but I loved the order of it and the way the practice glorified precision and suffering. To give in to the discomfort and leave early was failure. In black leggings and a sports bra, hair pulled back in a ponytail, sweat pouring out of me, I felt as if I were taking everything from the day—the stress of work, the noise of the subway, the stink of cigarette smoke and garbage coming in from the street—and depositing it on the mat. Through submission, surrender, there was peace. In a packed class one day, the man on the mat next to me tapped me on the arm. "Excuse me," he said, "I just have to tell you something." I looked at him. "I would consider you a really hot girl, except your elbows are really dry," he said. "You need to put lotion on them." Even in yoga class, I was an object that merited approval or dismissal based on the way I looked. I thought of my body as something that was functional—something to be pushed, if not punished.

So I continued pushing. My first year living in New York,

I ran the marathon—another accomplishment. Every so often I saw runners wearing neon-yellow shirts that read "Guide" on the backs; these runners, I learned, partnered with disabled athletes through an organization called Achilles. Passersby cheered when they and the disabled athletes they were assisting ran past. It was an act of kindness, and it made me think of my father, who had brought Reid out with us kids, knowing that Reid's own father, who was disabled, could not. In New York, a city that could be so hostile, to see people come together in the service of others lifted my spirits; it made me feel like I was not so far from home.

Not long after I ran the marathon, there was an open assistant job at *Sports Illustrated*. Given my lifelong interest in athletics, I applied. In the interview, as ever, I deployed my congenial Texas manners, answering every question with a polite "Yes, sir." I had been raised to do this, as had everyone I knew from back home; it was seen as a sign of respect for your elders, but I could tell the old-fashionedness of it made the man who would become my new boss uncomfortable.

After I got the job, during my first week, he pulled me aside. "Hey, just a heads-up," he said. "You gotta cut it out with the 'Yes, sir,' 'Yes, ma'am' stuff. It makes you seem subservient." He was right. I worked hard to strip it from my vernacular.

But this tendency to defer to authority was deeply ingrained. I had grown up in a culture where children were guilty until proven innocent; if a teacher called home about one of his kids, my dad's default response was "Go ahead and punish them. They can explain themselves when they get home." As an adult, I always made sure to toe the party line. I never wanted to rock the boat. Even after James, who had gotten a job on Wall Street and got married, I continued to socialize with him and his wife as if nothing had ever happened between us. I was committed to my game face, no matter how uncomfortable it made me. And as I made my life busy with my new job in a Midtown skyscraper, moving into a new fifth-floor walk-up with only one roommate instead of four, trying new restaurants, and going on dates with guys who told me they worked in finance without ever elaborating on what that meant, I felt like I was living a very cosmopolitan life—the kind of big, busy, grown-up existence I'd seen in magazines.

But in being so busy, I also felt like there was some meaning I was missing. The hours at my new job were long, even by my standards. I would find myself hunched over the fax machine at midnight, then stagger gratefully down to the bank of cars that waited on Fifty-first Street to take staffers who worked late back to their apartments. My mother had been diagnosed with breast cancer; she had a lumpectomy, and her prognosis was good, but there was so much uncertainty. Lizzie moved home to spend more time with her. She was a consummate caretaker, and she and my mom were deeply bonded from the years my mom had spent making sure Lizzie didn't fall behind. It was a familiar dynamic: I was achieving out in the world, while Lizzie had the space to be caring and to be with my mom. Life felt fragile, and I envied the time they got to spend together.

I went on dates with men with whom I had nothing in common, men toward whom I felt nothing more than a detached fondness. I tried dating men who were from Texas, thinking we'd connect over our home state. One took me on several dates filled with lovely conversation, but it never got remotely physical; one night, getting out of the back of a taxi, I came within inches of his face, hoping he would kiss me, but he fell backward, wriggling away from me. Years later, I would learn that he'd come out of the closet not long after we dated. Another guy arrived late to our date, street parking his Range Rover in front of the restaurant and throwing his briefcase down on the chair next to me. He looked over my shoulder throughout the meal, then, as we finished our entrées, announced that he had to get back to the office and left me with the check. The next day, he wrote to me asking if I'd like to go out again.

I no longer felt like Carrie Bradshaw. There were fewer Sunday brunches with friends from college now, and more work travel, worried phone calls home, and trips back for engagement parties, since many of my friends were starting to pair off and lead more domestic lives. I felt listless and confused. A friend recommended a therapist. Her only qualifications, as far as I could tell, were that her office was close to my work and she took my insurance. The co-pay was twenty dollars, which I could afford, and it felt like an appropriate thing for a young woman leading a fast-paced life in New York City to do—to go see a therapist—so I went.

The office was sparsely furnished, near Columbus Circle, with an Eames chair where the therapist sat and a large green potted plant on the parquet floor. She was a mousy woman with an impersonal demeanor; sitting in front of her, I felt only a vague curiosity about what I was doing here.

"Why did you decide to come see me?" she asked.

"I actually don't know," I said. "I don't really know what therapy's all about. This isn't a thing where I'm from." I hesitated. "I've been here two years and had a lot of bad dates, while my friends are starting to pair off. I feel like I'm going in circles. I'm starting to wonder—is there something I'm not addressing?"

Before she could respond, I began to sob inconsolably. I did not know why I was crying, but I could feel that there was a deep sadness within me—a loneliness, a fear that I was not desirable or worthy of being chosen. Whatever the game was, I was not playing it right. All I could do, in the moment, was cry, and so I did for the duration of the session. I did not go back.

Therapy, I thought, was not for me. I had always been physical and athletic, never someone who wanted to linger on feelings too long. Perhaps I was just a tactile-kinesthetic learner, someone who needed to move to process, instead of talking about things. Was that such a bad thing? Something needed to change, but I was convinced that therapy wasn't the thing that was going to change it.

Instead, I thought I needed to get out more—to *do* more. The problem wasn't that I was running. It was that I wasn't running enough. I was afraid that I would look back and regret having spent my whole life in an office building. My childhood had always emphasized the importance of community, and I knew the easiest way to feel good about myself was to do something for others.

I thought back to the disabled runners with the yellow jerseys and decided to sign up to run a marathon with Achilles. It would get me out of the office; knowing that this person would be waiting for me and needing my help would hold me accountable. And I would get to run.

.   .   .

THAT AUGUST, I WAS partnered with a man named Eddie, who had lost his vision as the result of a childhood illness. Now in his forties, he had attempted to run the marathon before, but training injuries had plagued him. After work, two friends and I would meet Eddie in Central Park, where we would take various routes to hit our training goals. Eddie held on to one end of a two-foot-long rope while one of us held on to the other end, running alongside him; another of us would protect him from the rear, while the third would cover him from the front. "Watch out, there's a pothole!" the runner in front would say, while others would call out to other runners or cyclists passing by, "Be careful—blind runner." In this way, we kept Eddie safe as he trained. It was the most useful I'd felt in a long time.

Not long after I started running with Achilles, I was in my cubicle at work when an email popped into my inbox from a man named John Griffin. He had heard through mutual friends that I was training with a blind runner, he wrote, and he wondered if he could join our group. I told him that he was welcome to run with us.

John had gone to the University of Virginia, too, a decade before me. He was tall, handsome, and confident—even in running shorts, a T-shirt, and socks that came up a little too high on his calves. He had already run five marathons, he said, and he was eager to talk team strategy with Eddie. Although he worked in finance, John wasn't a cocky Wall Street type; instead I found him as playful as a Labrador retriever, and just as disarming.

On a cool Friday evening in September, after finishing our run, I was sitting on a bench on Central Park South, retying my shoes, when John sat down next to me. "What are you up to this weekend?" he asked.

"Probably going out with friends," I said. *Is he asking me on a date?* I wondered. *Or just making conversation?*

"Girlfriends?" he asked.

"Girls and guys," I said. "Just college friends." I wasn't sure where this was going. I hoped he was going to ask me to do something.

"Have fun!" he said warmly. No invite. But I could tell he was gathering facts.

It was only a few weeks later that Eddie asked if John and I were dating.

"No," I said, "but he's great, isn't he?"

"Why not?" Eddie said. "Why aren't you dating? It's obvious that you like him."

"How can you tell?" I said.

"I may be blind," he said, "but I'm not blind."

I laughed. "I do like him," I said. "I like him a lot, actually. I can't believe I'm saying this, but I just know if I have one date with him, I'll marry him." I meant it. There was something powerful growing between us; whatever I felt for John I hadn't felt for anyone before. But I didn't want to ruin the congenial team atmosphere, since we were all training together. Besides, I had gathered that John was dating someone.

On 9/11, I watched the towers come down on a television in my Midtown office, which made the devastation feel as far away as Texas. It wasn't until I walked home from work through an empty Times Square, where I could see the plumes of smoke rising above the cityscape and fighter jets flying overhead, that it felt real. I sat in my shoebox West Village apartment, numb and scared. When I heard my phone ringing at the bottom of my purse, I fished it out and saw John's name on the caller ID. The cell towers had been so jammed that nobody could make or receive calls. I realized, suddenly, that John had become the person from whom I most wanted to hear, the voice on the other end of the line that I knew would be a comfort. I picked up. "John, I'm so happy you're calling," I said.

"I just wanted to check on you to make sure you're all right," he said. The world was crumbling, but as I sat on the floor talking to John, I felt that I was safe.

The night before the marathon, our running group went to dinner together. My mother, whose cancer was now in remission, came up from Amarillo, along with Lizzie. John and I danced around each other all night, as toasts were given and I handed out the T-shirts I'd made for race day. Later that night, my mom popped her head into my bedroom. "What a fun night," she said. "Is there something going on between you and that man?"

"What man?" I said.

"John," she said.

"No, Mom," I said, half blushing. "There's nothing going on." I was downplaying it because nothing had happened, and I didn't know if anything ever would.

Eddie finished the race, which was a cause for celebration. But in the weeks that followed, I had the blues. I missed spending time with the team, the endorphin rush of the runs, and having a purpose that didn't involve marketing decks and Monday-morning meetings. Yet more than all that, I missed seeing John.

A week later, the phone rang. It was John. "I have an event in the city next week," he said. "I'm wondering if you would come as my date."

. . .

THE EVENT WAS A black-tie gala in Midtown to raise money for Parkinson's, the kind of fancy party I'd see pictured in the glossy magazines I bought at the bodega on Horatio Street; John was on the board of the foundation, and he had a table. I left work early so I would have time to get my hair done and run home to change, then get back uptown for the gala. I wanted to try a chic new look, so at the last minute, I decided to have my hair styled in tight, coiled curls—something I had never before attempted. It looked like I'd been electrocuted, and I regretted it immediately, but it was too late to undo.

By evening, there were torrential rains. I stood on Perry Street in my black jumpsuit with my coat over my head, desperately trying to hail a taxi to no avail, then trudged to the subway so I wouldn't be late. Maybe I'd get lucky, I thought, and the rain would wash my curls into waves.

John was waiting patiently for me in the lobby, looking dapper in a black tuxedo—a far cry from the last time I'd seen him, in his yellow Achilles jersey at the marathon. I was wet and disheveled, harried from the journey uptown. But he was gentlemanly. "Wow!" he said. "Your hair! I almost didn't recognize you." He grabbed my hand. "I'm so glad you're here. You look beautiful." As he led me through the ballroom, I could feel that people were looking at me, curious to see whom John Griffin had brought as his date.

At the table, I looked for my name tag; I was seated to the right of John, and to his left was a famous supermodel. I did a double take at the name tag. *Oh, great.* When she sat down, her hair was in the exact same style I had attempted, but she was actually pulling it off. And yet, to John's credit, he barely glanced at her all night. He was so focused on me. I felt as if I were the only person in the room.

When the night was over, he whisked me into the black car that was waiting for us outside. "I can take you home," he said.

"It's all the way downtown," I said.

"I don't mind," he said. "It's more time with you." He reached for my hand. It fit perfectly in his.

JOHN'S PHILOSOPHY IN ALL things—business, romance, deciding what to order for takeout—was this: Long no, short yes. What this meant was, if he found himself deliberating, equivocating, and questioning a decision—if it took him a long time to reach a conclusion—the answer was no. If he quickly and definitively committed to something, the answer was yes. He trusted his instincts. With him and me, it was a short yes.

From the beginning, dating John felt different. When he said he would call, he called. When he said he would be somewhere, he was there. With men, there had always been danger: danger that I would fall short of their expectations in some way, fail to meet the ferocity of their desire, or that they would want more than I was comfortable giving. With John, the safety I felt was absolute.

John had made a lot of money in the markets, but his temperament was different from those of the other finance guys I'd known; he was kind, patient, and wise. He had grown up middle-class in Westchester, where his mother was an English professor who had written books on Shakespeare; he still loved the theater and read voraciously. The first time I opened his refrigerator, it contained a single jar of cherry jam, chicken salad, and a package of toasted raisin crackers. I never had more than half a burrito in a takeout container in my fridge, so I was relieved that he wouldn't expect me to be much of a cook. On the Fourth of July, after we'd been dating for a little less than a year, we took a trip down to Virginia. After a dinner of hot dogs and watermelon on paper plates, my hair still wet from the pool, just as it had been from the rain on the night of our first date, he proposed.

It was easy to love him and to be loved by him. After running so many long distances, I felt I had run into the right arms—of this good man, who treated me as an equal. With John, I felt as though my life could finally begin. I had been chosen, and not by just any man but an extraordinary one— one who was curious and funny and focused, whom the world recognized as successful. He would take care of me, and I of him. Wasn't that all that had ever been expected of me? The way it had felt to finish the marathon was how it felt to know that I had John, and he had me. Now I could rest.

EXCEPT I COULDN'T. I didn't know how. Sometimes it felt like something was chasing me—a monster of some kind. I couldn't see it, but I knew it was there. Every so often it would make its presence known.

Lizzie put together a video of friends and family sharing memories about my childhood, which she showed at a dinner days before my wedding. The stories people told in the video were fond, some gently embarrassing or cringeworthy. But when our longtime babysitter appeared on-screen, chuckling, I felt my stomach drop. I knew what she was going to say. She was going to reveal a secret, something that only she and I knew. I squirmed in my seat, eyes locked on the screen. She laughed as she recalled how I'd hidden my worn underwear in secret places around my room after I'd gotten my period. Out of the corner of my eye, I caught a glimpse of Lizzie burying her laughter in a napkin. I felt that feeling again, the one from the auditorium at the awards ceremony, the one I'd felt with James—like I was disappearing, or as if this were happening to someone else.

As the video ended, I gathered my senses, bolted from my chair, and beelined for the bathroom, face flushed. I felt so exposed—had that really just happened? Lizzie and my mother caught up with me in the hallway.

"It was so fun pulling all of those people together," Lizzie said. "Did you like the video?" She was smiling good-naturedly; I knew she had no malice. If anything, she was proud of herself for having assembled all those stories from my past. Then she saw my expression.

"I never want to see that video again," I said. I could hear the cold, contained fury in my voice. Her face fell. I turned on my heels, went into the bathroom, and took a few deep breaths, alone, trying to regain my composure.

How could I return to the party and continue making small talk with random cousins and uncles who were in town for the wedding? It was humiliating. But I couldn't let anyone see that I was rattled; I refused to be the girl who couldn't take a joke. I took the feeling, stuffed it down, and went back to the party.

It was strange. Until I saw that video, I had forgotten that I'd ever done that—that I'd hidden my underwear. But at the mere mention of it, all the memories came flooding back, and with them a deep shame. A tell I couldn't yet see.

. . .

SO I KEPT RUNNING, running every chance I got. I ran like my survival depended on it. I ran like I was in danger.

Running felt like the only space where I could control all the variables—the time, the pace, and how hard I pushed my body. But I couldn't control my memory, or where it wanted to take me. In my mind, I found myself transported back to Amarillo; the road in New York City would transform, becoming that old footpath that wrapped around the middle school.

I ran faster and faster. But there was always something nipping at my heels.

3. MIRRORS

People often told me that I had the perfect life. Every time someone would say that, I would look over my shoulder to see who they were talking to; certainly, I felt, they couldn't be talking to me. Even though perfect was exactly the thing to which I had aspired for so long, to hear it said out loud didn't feel right. "Perfect?" I would say, deflecting. "I don't even know what that means."

But I understood why they would think that. From the outside, at least, after I married John and we began building our life together, things did seem "perfect." I was athletic, tall, and blond. John was successful and respected in his career. I got pregnant easily and gave birth to a healthy baby boy, my son Jack. A baby girl, Grace, followed, then my daughter Gigi, and last, my youngest son, Julian. Four children—two girls and two boys, just like the family in which I myself was raised.

It was an abundant life, a beautiful life, a life in which I knew there should be no real complaint. And yet, and yet, and yet.

When did I begin to know that I was hiding something? I could not say. I cannot find a precise moment in my memory when the façade began to crack. All I know is that I became aware that there was something within me—something unexplainable, something deep, but something that I couldn't touch; a thing for which I lacked language. It was always there. It nagged at me with gnawed edges. I felt it in moments of pause, rare as they were. In the morning when I rose and went into the bathroom in my robe, barefaced, I found it was difficult to look at myself in the mirror. I felt so detached from whom I had once been, the little girl who had done cartwheels on the brick wall outside my house. When had I stopped doing cartwheels? I couldn't remember.

So I did what I had always done: I kept running. I ran on my honeymoon, on a treadmill in a hotel gym. I ran when I was pregnant, and then as soon as I got the green light from my doctor to run again after giving birth to each of my children. I ran with one child in a stroller, then somehow managed to run with a double stroller.

LIFE WAS BUSIER THAN ever as a parent of four small children. But that was good, wasn't it? Even the governor of Texas when I was growing up, Ann Richards, who had a quick tongue and a beehive hairdo, said so: "If we rest, we rust," she'd famously quipped. It was advice I'd taken to heart.

For the better part of a decade, I was nursing a baby, carrying one toddler, and trying to ready another for admission to a preschool that would, as it had been explained to me by other moms on the playground, determine their fate. I dragged strollers out of the backs of taxis, sat in ballet classes, and juggled naptime schedules. I sourced Halloween costumes, elaborate Easter baskets, and thoughtful Christmas gifts. Anytime there was an opportunity for me to demonstrate my commitment to being an exceptional mom and community member, I wanted to be the best at it: There was no end to committees and benefits and end-of-school picnics, birthday parties requiring elaborate cupcakes, and athletic events in need of juice boxes. I was fortunate that we could afford childcare, but with no family in New York to help me, I felt that the health and happiness of my family rested solely on my shoulders. I wanted people to see me as a good mother by the way my children behaved and appeared; after all, they were a reflection of me. It did feel, at times, that I was doing more things *for* my children than *with* my children—things that had no bearing on my relationship with them, that they would never know I'd done—but such were the rarefied problems of a Manhattan mom. And for the most part, from the outside, it looked glamorous: I loved bringing my family from Texas to New York so I could share with them this fast, exciting life I'd built. It felt like another achievement, to run them through my New York City paces, and I wanted to be seen for it.

Yet as life marched on, I felt my anxieties begin to calcify. I had always been tightly wound, but I found that increasingly, my nerves could be triggered unexpectedly. John was patient and understanding, and yet the source of my panic often seemed to bewilder both of us. I had long been claustrophobic; ahead of a long flight, I would seize with dread anticipating the lack of control I'd feel flying through the air in a confined space. John would hold my hand, gauging my stress level by how sweaty my palm was. I reasoned that it was probably because my mother's brother had died in a plane crash when he was twenty-one, but the fear was paralyzing.

At a routine dentist appointment, I tried to tell the dentist that I was in pain while he was filling a tooth, but he wouldn't stop. Instead, he pressed the palm of his hand down on my left shoulder. "You need to be still," he said. "I'm almost finished." I obeyed, tightening my hands into fists and willing myself to stay still as tears ran down my cheeks. The second he set down the drill, I ripped off the paper bib and bolted from the room and past the front desk, sobbing. The receptionist stared at me, jaw agape, unable to understand why I was so distraught. Out on the street, I couldn't catch my breath. I hunched over, gasping, with my hands on my knees.

Once, John found me stretching on a yoga mat at home. "I like what I see here," he said playfully. "You in those tight pants."

"Oh, you're funny," I said.

"What if I took this," he said, picking up a yoga strap, "and kept you here in this room with me?" He reached for my hands and fastened the strap around them. He was being playful, but I felt my body tense. As he began to pull the strap tighter, I felt the sudden, urgent need to escape. I pulled my wrists from the strap. "Stop," I said. "I don't like it." I could feel that I was in fight-or-flight, but I didn't want to embarrass him. I left him standing in the room alone, still holding the strap, looking confused.

He came to find me a few minutes later. "Are you okay?" he asked. "Do you want to talk about what happened?"

"It's fine," I said. "I'm not sure what that was."

"I want to make sure I didn't do something wrong," he said. "I would never want to make you uncomfortable."

"No, you didn't do anything wrong," I said. "I just had to get out. But I'm not sure why." We dropped the subject.

It was like my body knew something that I didn't. Over the years, I had thrown out my back many times; whenever it happened, I couldn't identify the source of the pain, only that it seemed to occur in times of particular stress. When my daughter Grace was an infant, my back went out while I was holding her, walking down the hallway. I collapsed, landing on my stomach, somehow managing to catch her in my arms as I fell to the floor. I would need surgery, but the thought of being put under anesthesia terrified me—a particularly unlucky phobia, given the toll all that running had taken on my body. Eventually, I had to have a piece of disc removed from my lower back, a place where I'd had chronic pain on the left-hand side. Years later, I had my right labrum reattached to my hip; seven weeks later, the same thing on the left. All in all, I was on crutches for over three months.

Sinus infections came and went for over a decade, but every time I went to the doctor, he assured me that every mom of young children was sick as frequently as I was. "Once they're all in kindergarten, you'll be home free," he said. It felt like he wasn't listening to me, but who was I to argue? He wrote me a prescription for yet another antibiotic and sent me on my way.

As the years ticked forward, my body kept telling me to slow down, but I just couldn't. I had two gears: fast and faster. I threw myself into physical activity, which had always been my escape, and spent months training for a triathlon. Swim, bike, run, repeat. In low moments I slapped felt bee stickers, like the ones my grandmother had always given me, on my helmet and shoes and bike; her memory kept me going. I would be at the YMCA pool at five thirty in the morning, then home in time to take the kids to school, leaving enough time to bike or run for an hour or two before officially starting the day. "What if you don't complete the race?" a friend asked. But the thought had never crossed my mind. Giving up was not an option.

With the triathlon, I had hoped to recapture the glory of my youth—all the volleyball matches I'd won, the tennis victories that had made my father so proud. But when I crossed the finish line into the arms of my children, surrounded by family and friends, I felt nothing. I waited for a wave of euphoria that never came. I woke up the next morning sunburned and dehydrated, aware only of an emptiness within me.

I NEEDED A NEW mountain to climb. I had been away from the workforce for nearly a decade, and now that my kids were all in school, I felt ready to go back to work. Over the years, I had been John's partner as he'd built his investment firm, watching from the sidelines but taking notes and honing my own instincts; now I wanted my own foothold in the world of business. I started small, making personal investments in founders of early-stage businesses, most of them female. Soon my days were filled with conference calls and board meetings; within a few years, things had grown to the

point that I started my own firm. I made sure my team knew
that they could reach me anytime, day or night. I had always
been sensitive about gender inequality: I remembered my
conviction that I'd have been a better class president than
Bradley Jones but also my certainty that he'd win only because he was a boy. Supporting female founders was a tangible way to empower women as they built businesses. Yet
more than that, I loved that the time spent focusing on others allowed me to avoid looking at myself. With my kids
growing up, it was nice to feel needed anew.

Yet at home, I was occasionally thrown by my own reactions to my children's behavior. I had never tested my parents' boundaries the way my kids seemed determined to test
mine. One night, my teenage son Jack brought home a girlfriend to our apartment, disappearing into his bedroom and
closing the door. This would have been a cardinal sin in my
childhood home. I stormed down the hall and flung his door
open.

"Mom," Jack asked incredulously, looking up from the
floor, where he and his girlfriend were crouched over his
computer, watching a movie, "what are you doing?" He had
grown into a charismatic, confident young man, rational like
his father. I must have seemed unhinged to him in that moment, but I couldn't explain why I felt like his being behind
a closed door had seemed like an emergency.

Later that week, when I was having dinner with a therapist friend, I admitted that I had done this to my son. "You
have to stop doing that," she said. "Where do you want him
to be intimate with girls—the park? You're modeling shame."
I thought back to how my father had talked to me about sex:
"Your mother was a virgin when I married her, and I expect
you to be the same." There had been no further discussion.

That's just the way it was in West Texas. Even though I had become much more progressive since moving to New York City, some vestige of those conservative southern values ran too deep for me to root out. One night, when I saw Gracie bolting stealthily for the front door, wrapped in a huge coat, I called her back so I could once-over her outfit. She was wearing ripped jeans, which back home would have been considered disrespectful or provocative. "Grace—" I started.

"I know you weren't allowed to wear them growing up, but it's not the eighties anymore!" she protested. "Everyone wears them now! It's not a big deal."

"Can you please just wear something else?" I asked. Gracie's friends, gathered at the front door, looking at the ground, pretended not to listen. But I knew they must have whispered about my ridiculous rules as soon as they got in the elevator.

ONE NIGHT, GRACIE CAME to my bedroom. "Mom, have you talked to Gigi tonight?" she asked. "She seems a little sad."

"About what?" I asked.

"I don't know," she said. "It has something to do with you. I think you should go talk to her."

At ten, Gigi was already verbally dexterous and loved to question authority; I suspected she'd grow up to be a lawyer. I went into her room and asked if everything was okay. Her demeanor was solemn as she collected herself to address me, sitting on the edge of the bed with her older sister next to her. I suddenly felt as if I were on trial.

"Mom," Gigi said, "I don't know how to say this, but I feel like I don't know you."

"Know me?" I said. "What do you mean?"

"I don't know," Gigi said. "I feel so disconnected from you."

Reflexively I became defensive. "Really?" I said. "After all that I do for you? My life revolves around trying to keep you safe and taking care of you."

"Mom, she's trying to tell you something," Gracie interjected. She was thirteen and reminded me of myself at that age: serious, driven, and focused. "We know you do everything for us. You make sure everything happens."

"But we don't feel like we know who you are," Gigi said. "You're nice, but you're not real. Do you have any idea how hard it is to have you as a mother? You do everything perfectly. You make everything look so easy. How are we supposed to relate to you?"

"Perfect is not my goal," I said. "I don't know what perfect even means." Yet even as I said this, I knew it wasn't true. Perfect had always been my expectation for myself. But hearing my daughter say it aloud bothered me, the way it always had when strangers told me I had the perfect life. I had indeed been raised to be perfect, but also not to draw attention to the quest for perfection. Perfection must look effortless. Being noticed for it invalidated it. The nuance was subtle but crucial—a distinctly southern twist on an old high standard.

Had I passed all that on to my daughters? The thought disturbed me.

"I'm just trying to be there for you," I said.

"You're here, but you're not here," Gigi cried. "Where are you, Mom?"

What could I say? How could I possibly explain? My daughters were asking me to participate in life, and in our relationship, in a way that I could not. There was a distance between us, and I was angry that I did not know how to bridge it.

I left the room, slamming the door behind me. In our bedroom, John was reading the newspaper in his sweats and a T-shirt. He set the paper down on his lap and looked at me. "What just happened?" he asked.

"I don't know," I said. "Gigi accused me of not being present. But everything I do I do for them. How can she not see that?" I sighed. "I never went through this when I was her age. I don't know what to do differently."

John took a long pause. "I know this is hard, but you're the adult. She's the child. I think you're the one who's going to have to do the work."

I threw my hands up and stomped into the bathroom. I didn't know what that meant. People often talked about this—"the work"—in a vague, wellness-minded way, usually without being specific about what it entailed. Therapy? I'd tried therapy. I wasn't sure what else to do. Now my own children were trying to hold a mirror up to me, but I could not bring myself to look.

So I kept running. I ran and I worked and I raised my children and ensured that I was too busy to feel much of anything. But sometimes, when I dove back into the swimming pool early in the morning to wear myself out in the chlorinated depths, I would scream at the top of my lungs, down at the very bottom of the pool, where I knew nobody could hear me.

MORE CRACKS APPEARED. I was on a trip, having dinner with three girlfriends, when one of them told a story about an inappropriate interaction she'd had as a little girl with an older man. Her description was vague, far from graphic. But I touched my face and realized that it was wet with tears. Another tell. "Amy?" one of my friends said. "What's wrong?"

Back in my hotel room after dinner, I found myself gripping the back of the desk chair, knuckles white, as I scanned the room for clues. I felt that familiar feeling again—exposed yet detached. I searched my memory. There was nothing there. I wasn't being honest with myself, but about what?

I pushed the feeling to the side. Whatever it was, I knew that I was not ready to face it.

Yet while I was shutting down, John was opening up. When I caught up with him the next day on the phone, his voice was warm and expansive. "Amy," he said, "I had an amazing session while you were away."

"Session?" I said. "Oh, that's right—your drug thing. How did it go?" John had become interested in psychedelic-assisted therapy, reading every piece of literature he could and eventually funding research into the subject. It was an area of personal interest for him: His father fought in World War II, and many of the clinical trials involving psychedelics were created to help veterans—a population who, he understood, had sacrificed so much yet often found themselves vulnerable upon their return. He followed the progress of clinical trials and their outcomes, and he'd undergone a few sessions himself. I had walls up about it, which was a testament to how deep my resistance ran: I had grown up in Reagan-era Texas, where drugs were patently off-limits, the domain of deadbeats and criminals. The message was received: My brain would be a cracked egg frying in a cast-iron skillet if I partook. My heaviest experimentation with mind-altering substances was pretending to take a hit off a joint at a party after graduating from college. I did not inhale, because I didn't know how.

"It was amazing," John said. "I'm learning so much about myself. I'd really like for you to meet Olivia, the practitioner I've been working with."

John had always been compassionate and levelheaded, but he had seemed markedly more open since trying psychedelic therapy. As long as I had known him, when someone at a dinner party asked about his childhood, he would say the same things. His mother was a theater critic with a late-night radio show, he explained; his father would accompany her, because she worked in an era when married women couldn't be out alone at 11:00 P.M. after reviewing a play. Sometimes he would tell the story of his parents interviewing Arthur Miller at the opening of *Death of a Salesman*. His father, John said, also ran the Westchester Youth Soccer League. If asked whether he had any siblings, John would say no.

All of this was true. And yet I knew there was more to the story. So it surprised me when, one night, not long after his first psychedelic session, we sat down at a dinner party and John answered the same old questions in a new way. "My father didn't have a job," he said. Coming out of him, the words sounded like a breath of fresh air. "He flew bomber planes in the Royal Air Force, and when he came back from the war, he suffered from PTSD, which prevented him from working. But that meant that I got to spend so much time with him. He was always there for me, like a stay-at-home dad." John didn't sound sad or embarrassed, and neither did his explanation. For the first time, he sounded grateful, at peace with the reality of his childhood.

When he was asked if he had any siblings, his answer, again, was different. "I did," he said. "Sadly, my sister was diagnosed with borderline personality disorder. She died by suicide when I was twenty-five."

He was so forthright and so clear. I had never heard him share this truth publicly. I studied him, wondering why the party line had changed, and so dramatically. It was a reminder that multiple stories could be true at the same time, that we select our narratives in accordance with how honest we want to be and how honest we can be with ourselves.

Whatever John had been doing had brought him home to himself—not in an abstract or touchy-feely way but as if he were simply more himself than he'd ever been before. I could hear it on the phone with him that day, just as I'd seen it over dinner.

"If it's important to you," I said, "of course I'll meet her."

OLIVIA LOOKED LIKE THE divine feminine incarnate— elegant, with long, wild auburn hair and porcelain skin, in a cotton sundress. I had expected a scene out of Burning Man, with crystals and sage; instead, she was disarming, polished, and wise.

Over dinner, Olivia fielded my questions. She had been in the psychedelic movement for decades, and she was gentle and knowledgeable as she explained her work to me. "So how long have you been a therapist?" I asked.

"Oh, I'm not a therapist," she said. "I'm a facilitator."

"What exactly does that mean?" I asked. "What are the credentials?"

She laughed. "A lot of experience."

"Experience with what?"

"Witnessing," she said, "as people find answers within themselves. I'm just there to facilitate an experience for them."

"And the experience involves drugs?"

"I call it medicine," Olivia said. "I always start with MDMA."

"Isn't that the same thing as Ecstasy?"

"Sort of. Ecstasy that you'd buy on the street isn't always the same compound, and sometimes it's contaminated with other things," she said. "Regardless, in a therapeutic session—which is quite different from a party or a rave—we use pure MDMA, and the setting is designed to orient you inward."

"So what happens in a session?" The table seemed to shrink as I found myself leaning in closer.

"I give you the first dose in the form of a pill," she said. "Then I'll give you eyeshades and play relaxing music. And I'll stay with you throughout the process to take notes on your experience, if you ask me to."

"Will you guide me through the session?" I asked.

"No," she said. "I'm not there to shape your experience, only to support you throughout. I won't interfere or prompt you in any way, so you can turn inward and focus on your own wisdom. And after, I'm here to help you integrate what you've learned."

"So what actually *happens* to the person? What do you feel?"

"Each person has a different experience," she said. "But I would describe it as meeting your most compassionate, loving self. Encountering your deepest knowing."

"And do you only do it once?" I asked.

"That's up to you," Olivia said. "Many people do multiple sessions, each spaced at least a month apart. But you'll know after your first session if it's something you want to do again."

"And what if you think there might be something there, something you've been hiding from yourself," I asked, "but you don't know what it is?" I rearranged my legs under my chair.

"Many people feel called to do this *because* they don't know why they feel stuck," she said. "They have tried everything and have nowhere else to turn."

"But if these drugs are so helpful, why aren't they legal?"

Olivia smiled. "Well, there's a complicated answer to that question that involves politics, racism, and the American obsession with morality, but long story short: Nixon and Reagan's war on drugs ended up criminalizing chemicals that had tremendous potential to heal and transform—even though psychiatrists were using MDMA experimentally in sessions in the seventies, long before it became popular on the street."

"What if I die?"

"You won't."

"Could we get arrested?"

"I don't think the authorities are all that interested in prosecuting people who take MDMA in a therapeutic context to improve their mental health," she said. "Given the ongoing research, it's going to be interesting to watch the landscape change over the next few years."

"How long is a session?"

"Six to seven hours, but it varies from person to person. It can last all day."

"Will I feel in control?"

"This medicine allows you to recognize that you don't need to be in control," she said. It was golden hour, half her face bathed in sunlight. Her words sounded like poetry. "It's a day with yourself—with the you that you've forgotten."

"So it's like rewinding," I said, "to the way you were before."

"It's not rewinding," she said. "It's rebecoming. You have always been your essential self. You just have to remember."

"What if I don't want to remember?" I asked. "What if I can't?" I shifted in my seat. "I've always believed in moving forward, not looking back. Can't I just keep going?"

Olivia was silent for a moment. "Of course you can, if going like this feels like your best life," she said. "But if there's some part of you that feels that something is missing, then no. I can only tell you what happens to people who run from pain: They never actually live." There was no judgment in her voice, only tenderness. "We don't recognize how much we carry our experiences in our bodies. If something is coming up"—she looked at me—"it has to come out."

Her words carried a heavy weight.

John didn't say much during dinner, allowing me to ask all my questions without interjecting his own experience. Finally, toward the end of the night, he gently touched my arm. "Amy," he said, "should we let Olivia go home?" It wasn't until I was walking her to the door that I realized she had never asked me if I wanted to schedule a session.

Getting ready for bed, John and I were brushing our teeth next to each other in the bathroom. There was a connectivity in the room, a charge between us. "That was great," John said. "I really wanted you to learn more about what I've been experiencing. It seems like you really connected with her."

He set down his toothbrush.

I turned to him. "I want to work with Olivia," I said. "I'm ready."

HOW DID I KNOW that this was what I needed to do? Even now, I don't really understand it. I just knew that I had built up walls, and I did not know how to tear them down. I knew that I was tired of running. And I knew that I could not hide in the vastness of the life I had built any longer—a life so big that I'd disappeared in it.

I had satisfied every expectation that the world had imposed upon me, met every demand that was made of me. I went to a good school, got a good job, married a good man, built a good business, created a good life for myself and my four children. Hadn't I done everything right? Hadn't I tried so hard to be perfect? I had chased validation from the world, and the world had granted it to me. But I'd never really felt it. I'd felt a void inside for years.

And now? I was blistered, run-down, exhausted. Incapable of rest. Terrified to stop for fear of what might emerge from the shadows. That night, brushing my teeth next to John, I realized I simply could not keep going like this. I believed that the pain of maintaining the status quo was greater than the pain of facing whatever it was I had been trying to outrun. For the first time, I could see a different path.

THE DAY OF THE session, I was anxious. "There's something I can't face," I told Olivia. "I know something happened to me, something I'm talking around. But I don't know what it is. It's like I can't remember. Or maybe I don't want to re-member."

Olivia looked unfazed. "Don't worry," she said. "I'll be with you. Whatever it is, you can handle it."

I held the pill for a long minute, looking at it. *Can I do this?* I wondered. I was taking an illegal drug with an unli-censed therapist to do—what, exactly? But I trusted John, and I trusted Olivia, and finally, I was going to trust myself. I swallowed the pill and put on an eyeshade. Then I sat in darkness, waiting. "How long does it take for it to kick in?" I asked. I could hear her moving a speaker around the room, the gentle sound of Spanish acoustic guitar playing in the background.

Olivia answered, confident. "About thirty minutes," she said. "Just breathe."

I FELT MY HEART pound in my chest. The rush of adrenaline. There was no turning back. I had taken the pill. Now I just had to get to the finish line. My system activated. It was just like running, like the route around the school I'd taken all those times. "How many loops did you do today?" my dad would ask. Because that was me—always running, running in a circle, right back to where I started.

Isn't life funny that way? You start off running from something, the point where it all began, and then, as it ap-proaches on the horizon, you realize that you haven't been running from it at all.

You've been running toward it.

.   .   .

JUST FIVE MINUTES IN, I sat up.

"Olivia," I said, "why is he here?"

"Who?" she said.

"Mr. Mason," I said, "from my middle school."

SUDDENLY, I REMEMBERED.

II. REMEMBERING

4. BATHROOM

The first thing I remembered was my head hitting the wall. Mr. Mason's hand was on the back of my head, pushing me up against the yellow tile in the bathroom of the middle school. Then I heard a *clang!* as his belt buckle hit the floor. The belt was brown leather with a gold buckle, and when I looked down at it, I realized: *I am in trouble.*

"Is everything we see real?" I asked Olivia softly. I reached for her hand. She was wearing a charm bracelet made of old coins. I gripped her wrist, clutching the coins as a reminder that there was something solid I could hold on to. "I don't think it can be real," I said.

"Stay with it," she said.

It was as if a film were playing inside my head, or rather, like I was the only person in a theater, watching a movie projected up onto the screen from the front row. I was not my younger self; I was adult Amy, conscious and aware, but I was being shown a vivid scene from my own life. It was familiar to me, this scene; I knew that I had lived it. Strangely, I did not want to turn it off. I could feel that it was important, this thing I was witnessing. Immersed in the session, I lost all track of time.

I saw myself on the floor, on my stomach, and he was stepping on my back with his cowboy boot.

"I must have made this up," I said out loud to Olivia.

My back was bare. Where was my shirt? I was twelve years old.

"This couldn't have happened to me," I said.

The rounded heel of his boot dug into the left side of my rib cage. I felt it in the same place where I'd had pain for years. I didn't move. I held my breath.

"Maybe I saw this in a movie," I said.

I looked around the bathroom. I knew every inch of that place. Even the divot in the sink that held the soap was familiar to me. The handle that would turn to open the window inward, directly opposite the door, which was closed and did not have a lock. The green stall and the gap between the bottom of the stall and the tiled floor. The toilet paper holder on the right-hand side of the stall.

"What is happening?" I asked Olivia. "I can't make it go away."

His hand was on the nape of my neck, pressing my head against the wall.

"I wasn't scared of him," I said. "I'm not scared of him now." A feeling had begun to slowly bloom inside me. A weight on my chest, but one of absolute security and truth. The place I had gone to had no fear, no insecurity, no doubt.

It was the place where my most essential self lived. I stared at the memory. It was all happening in real time.

"He was one of the good guys," I said.

In the memory, I was sitting on the toilet in the middle stall, facing him. I felt myself start to pass out, and as I slipped off the toilet, I remember thinking that I could grab on to the toilet paper holder to the right of me as I fell to the floor.

"He was always around," I said. "He cared so much about me."

He grabbed me by my left arm and pulled me along the floor to the middle of the bathroom. I saw the outline of his body moving, the crease in his pants at the knee, those cowboy boots, cappuccino-colored leather. Some part of him was always in motion, and I scanned his body from the ground up, watching the way he raised his arm or bent his knee.

"How can this be real?" I asked.

His foot was on my back again.

Then, a familiar memory—one I'd recalled so many times before, repeatedly throughout my life. I was walking down the hallway, and he stopped me, smiling. "We all know you're the real leader of this school," he said. I felt so special that day. He saw me for who I wanted to be.

"Mr. Mason," I said out loud, "thank you for seeing that in me, even though I didn't win."

And suddenly it was Navarro Day, the highlight of the middle-school year. My date was Bradley Jones, the boy who had beaten me to become student council president. I was so happy to be on his arm, even just for the night; I wished he liked me, that he wanted to kiss me, but he always had eyes for other girls.

"I asked Bradley to be my date," I said. It was a Sadie Hawkins–style dance, where the girls asked the boys. I was wearing a poofy dress with shoulder pads, in a bold floral pattern, made of fabric so thick it felt like wearing a curtain. I had borrowed it from a family friend. It was the first time I'd put on a fancy dress, and I loved the way I felt— ceremonial, important.

But then I was in Mr. Mason's classroom. It was early evening and still light outside. The frilly dress was pulled up over my head and I was bent over a desk while he was raping me from behind. I could feel the weight of the dress over my head, blotting out the light.

"This doesn't make sense," I said. "When would I have been alone at the dance?"

Next I was in the girls' locker room, with my hands on the metal locker, bent over at the waist. He was behind me. I felt the cold metal under my hands as he moved back and forth. I stared at the horizontal slats in the locker door.

"Could I be making it up?" I asked. But I knew that I wasn't. I was just trying to build a trapdoor in the scene, looking for an out. The fact of these memories was almost leaden, as if it were weighing down my body. I felt it in my chest cavity, the certainty of this deep truth, and I sighed heavily.

"I am going to tell him," I said, "*I know what you did to me*. I will ring his doorbell. Him in his fucking khaki pants. Always looking at me." I saw myself going into the bathroom and then leaving it, feeling numb.

Suddenly I thought of my daughters. "Oh my God," I said. "My girls." Gracie was thirteen and Gigi was ten. I felt a visceral need to protect them. Was I doing enough to keep them safe? "I can never let them be alone with anyone."

My memory turned back to the auditorium. Coach Taylor was talking about the recipient of the award. "This student works harder than anyone in her class," she said. "She is the teammate that lifts everyone up, she uses her body to accomplish extraordinary things, and above all, she is kind. She will go on to achieve greatness." I had wondered who it was. And then she called my name. Mr. Mason must have been in the auditorium, rows behind me. I could feel his eyes on the back of my head.

This memory was clearest of all—I knew it so well. I'd run through it in my mind a million times. I was crying, and so was my father. My mother was hugging me. I stood in the aisle, holding the award. I looked at my father's tears. And in a flash, I felt the edge that had been in this memory my whole life, that I had never understood before.

There was a brief moment, seeing the tears in my dad's eyes, watching him cry, where I wondered if he knew what was happening. He hadn't, of course—he was crying because he was happy. But the stickiness of the memory wasn't only because of his pride. It carried such a potent emotional charge and had remained with me all those years, because in that moment, I thought maybe I had been found out.

But I hadn't. Nobody knew. Instead, the world saw me how I wanted to be seen: as a leader. *The real leader of this school,* just as Mr. Mason himself had said. That memory, receiving the award, confirmed that if I just kept on achieving, nobody would ever have to know the truth. This was how I could continue hiding.

I had always thought back to that memory and felt confused. It had been exhilarating to be singled out, to be recognized. But I had also felt strangely detached, more numb than proud. I never knew why. Now, holding Olivia's hand, my adult mind lending insight to that childhood memory, I saw it clearly for the first time. I thought of that sweet girl, my barely-thirteen-year-old self, standing alone in front of all those people, being given an award, and the fear she felt on that stage. She couldn't be proud of what she'd earned through her hard work and kindness, not when she was so afraid people would discover her secret. I put my hand on my heart. The tenderness was almost unbearable. I felt profound compassion for that little girl—me—and all she'd endured. The warmth and sweetness and beauty reminded me of the way I'd felt that day in the sea in Ibiza—a perfect day, bathed in sunlight.

A weight I'd been carrying forever slipped off my shoulders. It was the first time I had ever been honest with myself about what happened. I did not feel any shame. I was free, free as I'd been as a girl doing cartwheels, free as I had been riding my banana-seat bike through the brick-lined streets of Amarillo.

"Oh," I said simply, realizing, "I did nothing wrong." Then I repeated it. "I did nothing wrong." I exhaled, accepting it. "This all happened."

I had been holding on to my denial like a life raft for so many years, certain that if I let go, I would drown. It was only once I finally did that I could allow the truth to take shape. And now, fully submerged, I found that I could swim—that I was just fine in these waters. Transfixed by the beauty and the horror of what I had been afraid to see from the surface, I wondered why I had waited so long to dive into the deep end. The only thing that had been waiting for me there was myself.

. . .

EIGHT HOURS LATER, LONG after the sun had gone down, the warmth of the medicine fading away, I took the eyeshades off, adjusting to the dim light. First I looked at Olivia. Then I pulled my hair up into a messy bun. I slumped over and buried my head in my hands. I felt as though an eighteen-wheeler truck had been parked in front of my house for as long as I could remember, emitting a low, polluting hum and blocking out the daylight. Now, as it drove away, leaving only peaceful silence and sunlight streaming in, the calm was disorienting. I didn't miss the noise, but I also didn't know how to live without it. Part of me wanted to jump onto the back as it drove away.

"How will I tell John?" I asked. "This will destroy him." There was no part of me that feared he would see me as damaged goods; I knew his love was unconditional. It was that I felt his love for me so profoundly that I did not want to hurt him by revealing my own pain. We shared everything with each other; irrationally, I felt like I had been keeping something from him, even though I had been keeping it from myself too.

I looked down at the floor. "Olivia, can you go get him?"

An eternity passed and then I felt him sit down beside me. I could not look him in the eye. I felt devoid of any emotion. I just had to say it, even though I knew that once I did, I would never be able to take it back. I held on to it for one final second before life changed forever, then I spoke.

"John," I said clearly, "I have to tell you something. I was abused by a teacher as a child." To say it out loud was both the most anguished and the most liberated I had ever felt. They were the most important words I had spoken to him since I'd said "I do" at the altar. The glass case of denial had shattered.

He paused for a long time and exhaled heavily. Then, slowly, he reached for me. "Amy, I'm so sorry," he said. He said more words, but I couldn't take them in; all I could hear was the grief in his voice.

John took my hand and led me into our bedroom, where he pulled the covers back so I could crawl into bed. It was late, and I was exhausted, but I could not sleep. Instead I lay awake, reeling. *Is my entire life a lie?* I wondered absently. *How am I going to recover from this?* As my awareness began to sharpen, some practical machinery appeared that I could grab on to. *What am I going to do now? How do I move forward? How will I get out of bed tomorrow morning? Will I ever eat again? How will I sleep? How will I survive? Is this a bad dream that I'm going to wake up from?* I had no answers, only more questions. Then—

"Can I help you into the bath?" I looked over to find John, his face etched with concern. I could see dawn peeking in from behind the curtains. I nodded gratefully, and he walked me to the bathroom, turning the faucet.

The sound of the water filling the tub had always given me permission to take a deep breath, an acknowledgment that it was safe now to unwind. This was the same tub where I'd taken baths with all my babies, the same tub I'd filled with buckets of ice to relieve my aching body after long training runs. But now all I could think about was how this was my first bath after my life had changed forever, a baptism in my new reality. The person who had taken all those baths was gone. I was someone new.

How had I not known? My memories of childhood were so crisp; even something as mundane as a bathtub like this one could trigger a host of images, sharp as photographs in my mind. There was the time Rachel and I shared a hotel room on the fifth-grade school trip to Washington, D.C., chaperoned by my mother and her best friend. I could recall with utter clarity the shock of pulling back the shower curtain to find them in their pajamas in the tub one night after we had come back from a monument tour, a half-drunk bottle of champagne smuggled upstairs, smoking cigarettes, crying with laughter. "Mom!" I said, stunned. "It looks like you're having fun."

She giggled. "Let's not tell your father about this," she said. "I promise I don't smoke."

Just as vivid was the occasion, around the same time, one of my siblings got the chicken pox. Back then, it was typical to put all your kids together so you could get the whole thing over with, so my siblings and I spent several weeks in and out of the bathtub, the water turning pink from the calamine lotion caked onto our little bodies. One year we even took a photo for our Christmas card in that tub. We were still young enough that all four of us could fit, covered in giant bubbles and grinning toothlessly.

I had submerged myself in so many bathtubs, in motels from Albuquerque to Austin, traveling for tennis and volleyball tournaments as a young athlete. I could see them in my mind's eye, those bathrooms, semiclean under institutional light fixtures, in tired rooms with faded accent pillows and Gideon Bibles in the nightstand, in chain hotels with rubber plants in the atrium and a complimentary continental breakfast, and I could remember all of them, those spaces where I'd allowed myself a few hours' rest before continuing to wear my body out.

How was it possible that I could remember all those bath-

rooms but had forgotten the one where something so horrific took place?

I had a *great* memory. I knew everything that had happened to me. Right?

I lay in the water, in silence, looking around the room,
searching for answers. I knew that John didn't have any. He
stood in the corner, his head hung low, one foot crossed over
the other and a hand resting on my vanity, balanced on a
delicate tightrope. I suspected he didn't want to take up too
much space, but he also didn't want to leave me alone. On
the edge of the tub, next to an expensive black candle I always thought about lighting but never did, was a milky white
bar of lavender soap. I had upgraded from Dove, the brand I
had long trusted because it was sold at the Toot'n Totum, the
soap I'd always packed in my monogrammed camp bathroom caddie from Joan Altman's. I'd used that soap for years,
then traded it in for something nicer, the way I'd done with
everything in my pursuit to make my life bigger, brighter,
and shinier—closer to some ideal of perfection that I couldn't
even define. There were so many invisible lines connecting
the girl I'd been to the woman I'd become, Texas to New
York, my past to my present.

I understood, suddenly, that everything was connected.
The choices I'd made in the life I'd built. The things I remembered and the things I could not bear to remember. In
a flash, all the pieces snapped together, and not just the
memories themselves but the significance of them; that is,
why they mattered. It clicked into place, crisply, like parts
that were designed to interlock. A jigsaw puzzle took shape
over my head, an awareness fusing, the way people say
something can suddenly dawn on you, as if I'd had the cor-

ner pieces assembled but not the full contents of the puzzle, and I had turned a little pile of cardboard fragments into a clear picture for the first time. Now it all made sense. I understood why there were things that I had remembered for so many years, that I had seen constantly, running on a track through my mind. Memories of Mr. Mason would come in like lighting a match, without warning and devoid of any emotion, then disappear from my brain—the flame extinguishing before I'd had a chance to attach any meaning to the memories. Finally, I knew what the memories *meant*— and I could hold on to them.

I saw myself running around the middle school, day after day, unable to look at it—turning away from the place where the abuse had happened.

I saw my disappointment when I lost the election to Bradley Jones, and then the prickling of surprise when Mr. Mason stopped me in the hallway that day. I felt so special.

He had known that I wanted, more than anything, to be seen as a leader. He had identified that need within me and he had exploited it. He had validated my desire to be exceptional, the same thing that had been nurtured in me by my parents and my school and my community—that I had come to believe was so important; he had taken this drive I'd had as a little girl, and he had used it to earn my trust.

I saw myself watching him pull out of the school parking lot, waving goodbye to me. That memory had replayed in my mind like a broken record, but I'd never known why it had felt so charged. Now I could feel my sneakers on the lip of the curb, that physical barrier that separated me from him.

I saw myself gripping the edge of the chair after my friend had recounted her own story of being violated as a child, knowing it had happened to me too, yet being unable to face it.

It was all right there. It always had been. I had just never been able to see it.

Rage bubbled up in me. I reached for the bar of soap, dense and slightly rounded at the edges. It felt good to grab something so solid. I cried out in anguish and fury, a mangled and desperate sound, and hurled the soap across the room. It hit the floor with a thud, skipping along the tile, leaving a thin trail of suds, and landing at the base of the sink, next to John's feet. He leaned over to pick it up.

"That's how he got to me," I said. "He told me I was special." I shook my head. "That's why I spent all that time alone in the school hallways. That's why he found me in the hallway to tell me he knew I was the real leader." I slapped the surface of the water with my hands, spewing the words out. "Oh my God, that's how he groomed me! I see how it all happened!"

John took my hand to help me out of the bathtub. I stepped out, wrapping myself in a towel. As I walked back into the hallway, I felt my body start to quiver, then give out. I fell to the floor, towel half covering me, shaking violently. I wailed like a wounded animal, gripping the carpet, trying to hold on to the solid ground underneath me with my hands while I kicked the wall with my bare feet.

"What can I do?" John asked calmly. I looked up and he was standing above me, and even though his face was so kind, the sight of a man standing over me in a bathroom was a too-familiar echo of something menacing.

"Can you come down here?" I sobbed. "Please sit with me and put your hand on me."

Slowly, he sank down onto the carpet next to me, as close as he could get. Gently he pressed one hand onto my lower back, where the towel was wrapped around me. I was still wet from the bath. "I can't get up," I said, weeping. "I can't move. I don't know what to do."

Minutes passed as he sat with me. "You don't have to do anything," he said. "You can stay here as long as you want. I'll stay with you. Just be here."

THAT FIRST MORNING, THE world was unrecognizable to me. I made my way onto the street, outside for the first time in nearly twenty-four hours. A doorman down the block greeted me, friendly as ever. I pushed wordlessly forward, my head down, eyes obscured behind sunglasses. Cyclists and joggers gathered at the entrance to the park, ready to take on the day. I sat numbly at a coffee shop, staring into my watery iced cappuccino with its cheerful red straw. I wasn't ready to face my life yet.

Back at our apartment, John handed me a blank journal that he'd had in a desk drawer, a navy blue notebook. "Journaling was important for me after my first session," he said gently. "It helped me get grounded and sort through what I was feeling."

I turned the notebook over in my hands. On the cover was embossed text that read: PLEASANT DREAMS. I would have found it funny if it weren't so painful.

I scribbled down only a few sentences the day after my session. "I lent a dress to a sweet girl, Claudia," I wrote. "Being kind and doing things for others created a distraction from what was happening to me."

Why was Claudia, a girl I'd barely known, the first thing I wrote about after recovering these memories? It was because there was another memory, one that had played repeatedly in my mind for years, long before the session with Olivia. Now, in a flashback, I saw it again: Mr. Mason was standing in the hallway by the cafeteria talking to Claudia. His hand was on her shoulder. I walked past, slinking behind them into the bathroom. I had never understood the significance of this memory, why it had stayed with me.

Now it made sense. On some level, I must have assumed it was happening to her too. The sight of them together made it real to me in a way that my own abuse could not be. Through the prism of Claudia, I had experienced the horror of what was being done to me. And in the memory, after I slid past them and through the swinging door, I stood in the empty bathroom with my hand on my heart and took several quick breaths. My chest was tight. I was panicked. My inhalations were shallow. I was so relieved he hadn't followed me inside.

There was another memory, from around the same time, that had always been with me. I was peering through the slats of the venetian blinds in my childhood bedroom as I saw a car pull up on our street. Claudia got out and walked up to the front door, carrying the dress I had loaned her in a thin, plastic dry-cleaning bag.

She rang the doorbell.

I hid in my room.

I was embarrassed for her.

I was embarrassed for us both.

I had always thought the feeling, that flush of shame, was because I was self-conscious that my family lived in a better neighborhood than hers. But was there more to it? I could not be sure. What if nothing had happened between Mr. Mason and Claudia, and instead I had projected what was happening to me onto her? Had I given her the dress in a subconscious show of solidarity because I believed she too was being abused? Or was I only thinking that now that my own abuse had been unearthed? It had all been so long ago. I wondered where she was and what kind of life she'd built for herself. Eventually, I thought, I would find her.

I thought about this, the gears of my mind turning as I tossed and turned in my bed, as the first twenty-four hours became the first forty-eight, as day turned to night and back again. I canceled everything on my calendar. It was the height of summer, and my children were busy with sports, camp, and friends. I knew they could withstand a few days of my hiding in my bedroom. I spoke only to John.

"When am I going to tell my parents?" I asked him numbly. It was late at night, and I couldn't sleep. "This will break my mom."

"I don't know," he said, shaking his head, "but I'm not sure if your dad can handle it." Would he even believe me?

ON THE THIRD DAY after the session, I dragged myself to the gym to swim in the pool, knowing that the water would bring me comfort, as it always did. As I crossed the surface, an image of a blue bandanna flashed through my brain. At first I couldn't place it. But as I stayed with the image, I realized that I'd seen it before—from Mr. Mason. He had used a blue bandanna to tie my hands behind my back in the middle school bathroom.

I swam faster, my freestyle propelling me across the pool. *What the fuck?* I thought. *How could I not have remembered that?* I thought back to John playfully tying my hands with the yoga strap all those years earlier, my seemingly inexplicable reaction. *How could I not have known?* I took a big gulp of air, dipping back below the surface.

Then I saw an open mouth full of teeth, like what a dentist would see staring down at a patient. And I heard Mr. Mason's voice.

"If you tell anyone," he said in a low Texas twang, "I'll rip your teeth out."

I gasped. Was it really possible that he'd said that to me? I remembered how I'd run out of the dentist's office in a panic, hysterical. I pulled myself out of the pool, feeling the muggy air hit my skin, and bolted for the locker room.

It wasn't until I got into the car with John that the pieces of the memory suddenly fused together. I saw myself on my knees in the middle-school bathroom, Mr. Mason's bandanna keeping my hands tied behind my back as he shoved his penis into my mouth. Then, in my memory, he was washing my mouth out with a bar of soap. "You come from one of the nicest families in town," he said. "No one will believe you." No wonder I had hurled that bar of soap across the room a few days earlier. The solidness of it, feeling its weight in my hand, had made it real.

The floodgates had opened.

An electricity surged through me, from the top of my head down to my toes.

"Why didn't anyone save me?" I screamed. "Why didn't anyone protect me?" I thrashed wildly, tearing at the seat belt. "I can't handle this!" My body jerked and convulsed involuntarily, my muscles seizing. There was so much rage pulsing through me, I could have shredded the seat belt into ribbons.

THREE DAYS LATER I was sitting across from Lauren, a fine-featured woman with chestnut hair and a warm but professional demeanor, who had come highly recommended by our family doctor. I was desperate for a lifeline, and Lauren—with her pedigree, medical credentials, and expertise in both trauma and psychedelic-assisted therapy—was it. Sensing that I was in extreme distress, she had cleared several hours for a consultation. I curled up, wrapped myself in a blanket, and started talking.

I told her the story of my childhood, and how my parents had raised me; about the culture of Amarillo, and how much had changed for me since leaving Texas. Lauren listened attentively, affirming my experience where she could. "It sounds like your parents loved you a lot," she said. "It also sounds like the expectations placed on you—from them, and from yourself—were incredibly high."

We'd been talking for more than an hour when I finally started talking about the memories I'd recently uncovered. I didn't cry as I recounted what I remembered. It felt good to say the words to another person, to get the images out of my brain. Yet as I talked, I could feel my own doubt beginning to slip in. The memories were so clear, the images so vivid. I could feel these experiences so viscerally in my body that they *had* to be real. But how was it possible that I hadn't remembered the abuse—not even one fragment of an image—for so long?

Wrestling with my doubt, I interrupted my own story to ask Lauren a question that had been gnawing at me: "Can you explain how memory actually works?"

She paused. "That's a great question, and I think I understand why you're asking it, so we'll talk more about that. But the fact is, scientists are still studying how memory works, even at the cellular level. I can explain some basic science that researchers agree on, but the reality is always more complicated."

"That's okay," I said. "I really want to understand." I loosened my grip on the arms of the chair.

"For starters, memory involves three phases: encoding, storage, and recall. First, let's talk about encoding. For example, just now, you were probably noticing some things about me, including what I'm wearing, but not every detail of that, right? The term 'encoding' refers to how different kinds of input are processed by the brain and converted into a neural code, which can then be stored. But only *some* of what's experienced—basically what gets your attention and is significant to you in that moment—gets encoded into your short-term memory, and your short-term memory only lasts about thirty seconds."

I nodded.

"But even after something's encoded in your short-term memory," she continued, "only *some* of that information will get stored in your long-term memory. What our brains tend to store is whatever was most salient to us in the moment. And, importantly, we never store *everything* about any experience."

I nodded again. "I guess that's why I only remember some pieces of it."

"Exactly," she said. "In any experience, there are both 'central details' and 'peripheral details,' but only the former, which are generally judged by the brain to be more important, typically make it into long-term memory."

"But how does that make sense?" I said. "If central details are stored in long-term memory, wouldn't you *remember* them? What happened to me was so significant, but I only just remembered it."

Lauren leaned forward a bit. "Well, let's talk specifically about what it means to 'remember' something. There's a difference between a memory that's *stored* and a memory that's *recalled*. You're right that stressful and traumatic experiences tend to be stored very strongly, as a part of your brain called the amygdala begins to release norepinephrine and cortisol—two hormones that burn central details into long-term memory. But—and this is really important—just because something is strongly *stored* in your memory doesn't mean that it will be *recalled* later, or ever. That's because storage and recall are *different* memory processes. Recall only happens when the *conditions* are right."

I paused, processing what she was saying. "How are you feeling about all of this, Amy?" she asked. But I wasn't sure what to say. Fragments of memory—a cold bathroom floor, a boot on my back, a silver-plated toilet paper holder—flashed through my mind.

"Keep going," I said. "This all makes sense."

"So when we talk about memory recall," she said, "we're often talking about the context in which it takes place. Those might be places or situations, but it can also be internal experiences—like an emotion that reminds you of something that you felt during a traumatic experience. There are also cues that facilitate recall. For childhood sexual abuse, a cue that triggers memory recall might be being touched or looked at in certain ways. For combat vets, it could be hearing a car backfiring or a helicopter overhead. For you, it may be worth exploring what finally enabled you to remember."

"It was the MDMA, right?" I said. It seemed obvious. "Why did it release this flood of memories?"

"Well, I think the MDMA was only a part of it," Lauren said. "MDMA can help a person feel safe and connected within themselves. It calms activity in the amygdala and releases oxytocin—a hormone that increases connection, trust, and the brain's capacity to learn and change. But you told me you felt truly safe with Olivia that day. Feeling so safe with someone can allow the recall of memories that were blocked out for so long. The fear, shame, and avoidance can all be relaxed, or even temporarily dissolved."

My own doubt was softening, but I felt acutely anxious as I thought about how others might react. "What if people think I was hallucinating?"

"It's important to remember that MDMA is not classified as a hallucinogen. It's been called both an 'entactogen'—because it enables a *touching within* that promotes introspection and reflection—and an 'empathogen,' because it can evoke deep empathy for oneself and others."

This didn't do much to reassure me. "Right, but couldn't these be false memories?" I said. "How can I trust myself?"

"Let's be clear—I'm not the arbiter of truth. But I have no reason to suspect these are false or implanted memories," Lauren said. "All of these memories arose organically. Olivia never guided you toward them, and they began even before the drug effects had set in." I nodded. She continued, "I think it might be important to ask how these experiences are showing up for you and how you are feeling them in your body. Even with the MDMA, you clearly didn't experience them as mere hallucinations. You describe them the way trauma survivors describe flashbacks—vivid sensory experiences—as though you were back in those rooms where the abuse took place."

"Olivia said it seemed like the memories were there just beneath the surface, as if they were waiting to come out," I said.

"Maybe just by virtue of deciding to take MDMA, you'd already decided you were ready to confront the past. So even before the drug effects set in, you were in a more open state psychologically," Lauren said. "You told me you knew there was a door locked inside you—that was why you were interested in having a session in the first place. The combination of MDMA and your relationship with Olivia may have helped you to open it further, so you could see and feel it all with less fear, less shame, and more compassion for yourself."

I nodded. What she said resonated. Still, I wondered aloud: "So why is it all only coming up now?"

Lauren took a deep breath. "That's a great question, and one I can't answer for you. I do wonder about how your relationships, even beyond the MDMA and your connection to Olivia, may have shaped your readiness to know all of this—to bring the trauma into your awareness, so you could begin the process of healing. You've talked about John, but you've also mentioned your daughters. How old are they?"

"Gracie is thirteen," I said. "Gigi is eleven."

"Have you thought about the role that they might play in the timing of all this?"

I took my own deep breath, pulling the blanket up around my face. "They're the same age I was when I was abused," I said. My eyes welled with tears. "I see so much of myself in them."

"It's not uncommon for women to begin remembering their trauma when their children reach the age when their abuse took place," she said. "We've been talking about memory recall, but based on what you've told me, it seems pretty clear that your *body* never forgot. You were physically shaking as you recalled the memories. Think about all the messages your body has been telling you—maybe for years—as you respond to various cues. And your *personality* never forgot, either—your perfectionism and people-pleasing, your inability to slow down. Even the decision to leave Amarillo and build a life in New York City may be important: It's been suggested that people with complex trauma prefer living in big cities, because the stimulating environment rewards their hypervigilance." I looked at her quizzically, and she continued: "Think about all the things you have to navigate just to get through your day in New York City." She smiled gently. "All of this is to say: Just because you couldn't recall your trauma on a *conscious* level doesn't mean it hasn't always been there, affecting your life."

"Is there some kind of medical diagnosis for me?" I asked. "Do I have PTSD?"

"Well, you certainly have symptoms of PTSD," she said. "Hypervigilance is one symptom. Ordinarily we diagnose PTSD only when those symptoms have significantly impaired someone's level of functioning, and your functioning is still remarkably high. But I think it's important to reflect on the many ways traumatic experiences can shape our lives and what it means to be affected functionally. We've become more trauma-informed as a society, so we are getting better at seeing now that people with trauma are more susceptible to mental illness, chemical dependency, and other chronic health issues—even if they seem to be doing well. What we don't always see is how the ambition of high-achieving people can be a trauma response. Sometimes the person who appears to have it together might actually need support."

"So what do I do now?" I asked. This was my biggest question, and the one I was the most afraid to answer. How was I supposed to go back to my normal life?

"This is the start of a much longer process, Amy," she said. "So let's meet again soon. In the meantime, try to be gentle with yourself. Try to take things slowly, and be conscious of who and what you're allowing into your system. You're still so sensitive—so vulnerable and raw. You'll want to be careful what you let in, and when. Be mindful of your boundaries." I nodded, not knowing exactly what "boundaries" were. Still, I was so grateful for her perspective and knowledge, and I wasn't sure I was ready for her to go. In these uncharted waters, Lauren felt like something sturdy— as solid as the string of coins on Olivia's wrist that I'd held on to during my session. A reminder that the wider world hadn't crumbled, even if it felt like mine was in pieces.

I TALKED WITH LAUREN for another hour, discussing what being "gentle" might look like. "Should I text you how I'm feeling?" I asked.

"That isn't necessary," she said, crisply but not unkindly. "We'll talk about it in our sessions."

"I text Olivia all the time—I even use emojis," I said, half joking.

Lauren smiled. "We're going to be working on boundaries, remember?"

After we parted ways, I felt a pang of something—nothing as pure as hope but maybe something like solace. I had found a resource, someone who would listen and understand. I had opened the lid to a container inside me that I was now ready to fill. I felt my chest expand.

At home, I went into the bathroom and turned the tap on the tub, watching as hot water flowed from the faucet. I filled the bath, stripped off my clothes, and got in, letting the warm heat envelop me once more.

Just because I was underwater didn't mean I was going to drown.

5. BOUNDARIES

In the darkness I felt after my first session with Olivia, my only kernel of hope was knowing that I still had my husband and my children. Those things could not be taken away from me; they were real and constant. Sitting at the dinner table listening to them talk about their days made me feel like I was still alive. As they ping-ponged stories back and forth, sounding happy and self-assured, I felt confident they hadn't endured anything like what I had as a child.

But then again, how could I be sure that they were safe? Zoning out at the table, I'd make lists in my head of all the people my children had been left alone with over the years. Was there any way to guarantee that they had been spared my fate? Were there clues I should be looking for? Was I paying close enough attention? Then I'd snap back into the present, to a dining room where Julian's spaghetti noodles were dangling off the side of the table and the dog was begging for a bite, and it all felt so normal, so benign, this ordinary domestic scene. How could anything terrible happen in this family I had built? *You just have to work twice as hard to keep them safe,* I thought. An old refrain with a new twist.

I was also preoccupied by doubt. I had no way to confirm what I'd remembered. There was no smoking gun, no physical evidence, no tangible proof. There had been no witnesses. I wasn't sure yet if I wanted to seek justice in some way, but I had this nagging sense that if I wanted to be seen as credible, I needed something more than memories, most of which had surfaced while taking an illegal drug. But how was I going to find evidence? What would constitute proof? All I had were these painful memories, playing on a loop; they were undeniable to me, but how could they be to anyone else? I felt I needed others to validate my experience.

I tried to keep some sense of normalcy, taking the kids out to the beach house where we'd spent so many summers. One afternoon, I took Julian to the water. My youngest son had grown into an energetic eight-year-old who never took off his soccer jersey and still carried a pink stuffed turtle around with him. The beach was mostly empty, the water lapping against our ankles, and he let me hold his hand as we walked. He was collecting shells, small cream and purple pieces that had washed up on the shore. "This is my one chance before they all disappear again," he said.

"I get it," I said. I understood the feeling. I'd begun to worry that everything I'd uncovered would somehow slip away again, get pulled back by the strength of the tide. I had to stay present in this moment while the memories were all fresh, instead of letting them drift away. I had to sift through what had surfaced.

As we walked, Julian picked up shells, handing them to me. "Will you please keep this one safe, Mom?" he asked. "It's really special."

"Yes," I said. "I got you." I held the shell tightly, but I held his hand tighter.

THE OTHER QUESTION THAT had begun tormenting me was this: How could I explain to the people around me what I had uncovered? Where would I begin? I knew that eventually I would need to tell my parents, but the thought was intolerable; the same was true of my siblings, particularly my sister Lizzie, with whom I had remained close. My children, too, I would need to tell at some point, but how, and when? Even telling my oldest friends felt daunting: People were dealing with their own lives, their own traumas, and I didn't want to unload on them without warning, but I also didn't want them to wonder why I suddenly seemed to be in my own world. Olivia had encouraged me not to immediately share with friends what I had discovered, advice that was echoed by Lauren and that I took to heart. "You owe it to yourself to sit with it all," Lauren said. "When you tell someone, it will take on new meaning. You'll be worried about their feelings and whether or not they believe you."

The strange thing was I found that I *wanted* to tell people. As much shame as I felt, telling people my story felt like a necessary corrective to the decades of silence. I felt like I needed to say it out loud, to own what had happened to me, no matter how difficult it was. A friend in whom I confided listened sensitively as we walked along the shore, the waves lapping at our feet. Not long after, she sent me a message. "I've been thinking about you a lot and I really think you need to talk to my friend William," she said.

"William?" I asked.

"Trust me on this," she said.

A couple of days later, William and I met to go for a walk together, on a sunny summer afternoon. He listened intently as I shared my story, stopping only when I mentioned a particularly graphic image. He put his hands up to his face.

"I am so sorry that this happened to you," he said, shaking his head.

He looked at the ground, pursing his lips. "I have to tell you, the same thing happened to me."

"What?" I said, incredulous. "With a teacher?"

"Yes," he said. "A teacher."

I stopped walking, just as he had a few minutes earlier. Now he paused a few feet ahead of me and turned back. I needed a moment to take in his admission. It was the first time since I'd remembered my past that I'd been met with a mirror. I had thought what happened to me was so uniquely violating, but of course there were other survivors, hiding in plain sight.

"William, I'm so sorry," I said. We resumed walking.

"He preyed on the fact that I needed a father figure," William said. "My mother was raising me on her own. Addressing what happened has been a long process."

"What did you do about it?" I said. "Where did you even begin?" We had come full circle, back to my driveway.

"After many years, I reported it to the school," he said. "They took the matter very seriously and hired a firm to do a thorough investigation. They even sent out a letter to grades above and below mine to ask if anyone else had memories of misconduct."

"And?" I said, nervously drawing circles in the gravel with the toe of my sneaker as I waited for his answer.

"Within a few months, several other survivors came forward," he said. "The teacher was eventually indicted. I submitted a confidential statement in which I told him what he'd taken from me, how he'd robbed me of my childhood. Ultimately he was incarcerated."

"William," I said breathlessly, "this is unbelievable. You were validated. He was held accountable. What an incredible outcome for such a terrible thing."

"Yes," he said. "I'm glad he's in prison, but it still feels like there's more for me to do."

In a flash, the road ahead felt clear. "This is what I'll do," I said. "I'll find other victims. They must be out there. I'll dig up all the facts, and then I'll be able to put this to bed and move on. Like you did." William tilted his head slightly, as if to caution me without words. "Your story has given me so much hope. I'm going to do this. I'm going to hold this man accountable. I want that same resolution you found."

William sighed. "But what I'm trying to say, Amy, is that healing is a long road." I looked at him, unclear. "On one level, it was satisfying to see my abuser convicted, and for sure it was the right thing to do, but there's so much more that I've had to do to process it all. There are two different but connected tracks: the work you do to process this for yourself and the external work you do in seeking justice. They both take time. Your first responsibility is to yourself. You have to take care of yourself, and the result of that work may be that others are helped, but first you have to address your own needs."

His invoking of my needs felt absurd. Needs? What were my needs? I needed details. I needed corroboration. I needed to find the evidence that would confirm my memories. I needed to make sure he could never hurt anyone ever again. And then I needed to throw the whole thing into the ocean and move on with my life.

"I can do both at the same time," I said confidently. "I'm so grateful that you've shared your story with me. How brave of you. The people in your life must be so proud."

"Well, actually, most people don't know," William said. "I haven't talked about it with anyone other than my family and my closest circle of friends."

"You haven't?"

"No," he said. "Even after all these years, I'm not sure I'm ready to do that. I'm still processing what happened. Besides, the school was able to protect my privacy. I never had to use my name."

I studied him. It was fascinating to me that William wanted to retain his privacy, when I felt like I needed to tell in order to explode the years of secrecy. It was clear there was no one right way to handle something like this. But hearing his story made me feel newly hopeful. The world would bend toward justice, would right itself to address what had been done to me.

I returned home to find John reading in the living room. "How do I find him?" I asked. I couldn't bring myself to say his name. I hadn't so much as looked him up online; the prospect of having to stare down a photo of him on the screen was unthinkable.

John considered it. "Is that something you're sure you want to do?" he asked.

I nodded. "I want to know everything I can about him," I said. "That's where I start."

"There's a firm I've used in the past to do background checks at work," he said. "Why don't I see if they can look into him?"

Just then, I heard footsteps in the hallway and looked up to see Gracie standing in the doorway. She was wearing ripped jeans, which I disliked—but when I looked at her feet, I saw she was also wearing a pair of high heels that I recognized as mine.

"Gracie," I said. "Are those my shoes?" Up until then, I'd only ever let my girls wear flats or a kitten heel; anything more than two inches felt risqué, a gesture toward womanhood that somehow seemed precocious.

"Mom, I'll bring them back," she said. "I swear. Please trust me."

Only weeks ago, I would have put up a fight. But now it seemed absurd that I had ever cared about the height of her heels. What was I trying to solve? Gracie was becoming a woman—so much so that she was borrowing my shoes. Did I really want to use this moment to criticize her?

"I do trust you," I said weakly. "Just put them back in my closet when you get home, okay?"

"I will," she said, scampering out. "Thanks!"

"And please don't walk through the grass," I said. "You know what happens to heels in the grass. It ruins the shoes."

IN MANY WAYS, I was sleepwalking. I'd checked out of my normal routines and responsibilities. I was in survival mode. I took meetings over video so I could stay out at the beach, and I left the house only to take brief walks around the neighborhood, keeping my head down to avoid looking neighbors in the eye. My memories—and the fact that I'd repressed them for so long—were disorienting in ways that defied language: How could I go on with anything that resembled my old life? And yet I needed more support than just John and Lauren. As I waited for the background check to come back, I knew that it was time to confide in the two friends who had known me the longest. I was desperate to know what they remembered and to find out if there was anything they might be able to help corroborate. I needed to tell them.

Rachel came over on a rainy summer morning. She and I had stayed close through college, sharing an apartment in New York for several years before we both married; we had raised our children in the city together until she moved back to Texas, although she still spent part of each summer on the East Coast. She was my oldest friend and a constant in my life—the very person I needed now. She held my feet as we curled up on the couch, and I told her the story of what I'd remembered. I could feel her energy coiled so tightly within her that the tension was almost unbearable. "I'm going to need some time to process this," she said. Her face was bright red, the same color it had turned when we were little girls walking into a roller-skating rink and suddenly our friends and family jumped out to yell "Surprise!" I looked at her sitting across from me and couldn't help but think about all the birthdays we'd shared. What had I been keeping hidden from her, and myself?

"Is there anything you remember about me during those years?" I asked.

"Oh my God, Amy," she said, shaking her head. Her eyes

were glassy, as wide as saucers. I could tell that she was try-ing to hold it together. "I don't remember any of this," she said. "Not the school. Not the classroom. Not this teacher. I do remember taking shop class with you so we could ask our dates to the dance. There was that kid Jason—remember him? The one who used to make throwing stars out of metal and hurl them at us across the room?"

"I can't believe he didn't kill us," I said.

"Yeah, well, that's the only thing that sticks out from those years."

"Do you remember when we were kids and we used to play with those horny toads?" I said. "They were the strang-est creatures, right? Flat and spiky, like little dinosaurs. They were everywhere when we were growing up, and they just disappeared. Do you remember them?"

"Of course," she said.

"That's what I was hoping this would be like," I said. "That I would say, 'Remember?' and somebody would just say, 'Of course I do.' But in this case, it's like I'm the only one who saw those frogs. And now they're gone, and I can't prove they ever existed."

Leaving, Rachel stood in my driveway with her shoulders slumped. She looked defeated. "I'm so sorry," she said. "I just wish I could do more to help you."

I played phone tag with Courtney for days; I had been begging her to come to visit from Austin, where she now lived, working as a middle-school counselor, but I knew she was busy with her two sons and work schedule. Finally, lying in bed one day with the covers all around me, I snapped and called her. "Hi!" she said brightly. "I'm just on my way to tennis—I wish you were here to play with me!"

"I have to tell you something important," I said.

"Let me pull over," she said. She could hear the gravity in my voice.

She was silent until I finished my story. "Oh, Amy," she said. "Amy, Amy, Amy." I could picture her in the driver's seat of her SUV, in her white tennis skirt, her blond hair in a ponytail, just the same as she'd been as my doubles partner in high school. "This makes me so mad. Oh my God. How can I help?"

Not long after we hung up the phone, Courtney began sending me texts. "I looked him up," she said. At first I froze; it was too close for comfort. But that's who she was: the academic, the investigator, always five steps ahead of me. "There's all these pictures of him with his gun collection. It's wild."

"Please don't send me any pictures," I said. "I don't think I can look at them."

A few days later we talked on the phone again. "I just want to go after him," she said. "This is not okay. You know I found Claudia, too?"

"You did? How? You and Rachel didn't even remember her."

"I know—that's why I had to look her up!" Courtney said. "Now she's living in—"

I cut her off. "I'm sorry, I'm just not ready to hear about it," I said. "But we gotta get you a job at the FBI."

AS RAW AS IT felt to share my story, I was relieved to have my two oldest friends in the loop, checking in on me and offering their support. My world felt like it had shrunk to the size of my bedroom. With my kids popping in and out of the house, I made a point of focusing what little energy I had on whichever child was home at any given moment, even if it was to make sure they were wearing sunscreen or to take them for ice cream. But outside of that, what I'd uncovered was all I could think about. I had been waiting two weeks for the background check to come back, hoping it would provide some comfort. Maybe it would contain some sort of smoking gun—that Mr. Mason was already a registered sex offender or something material to confirm what I'd remembered. I was getting stir-crazy.

On a muggy weekday morning, John and I got up early to go for a bike ride. It felt therapeutic to put on my gear and clip into my road bike. Just as I was fastening my helmet, John turned to me. "The report is back," he said offhandedly. "They didn't find much."

His casual delivery of what I considered earth-shattering news caught me off guard. "It's back?" I said. "And you haven't showed it to me yet?"

"Well, there isn't a lot to show," he said. "I just got it last night." He swung his legs onto his bike and clipped in. "Come on," he said. "Let's go."

Riding along the winding country roads, I could feel my pulse accelerating as anger smoldered within me. *How could he not have shown it to me immediately? Did he not understand that I was hanging on by a thread?* The contents of this report were everything to me. And all John could say was "They didn't find much"? When we paused at a street crossing, I whipped around to face him.

"I am so hurt!" I shouted. "You know how important this is to me, and you don't even tell me when it comes back? Are you kidding me? My whole life is hanging on this report!" Rage bubbled up. No one had defended me then, and no one was defending me now.

"Amy—" he said.

"Leave me alone!" I yelled, and I pedaled away from him as fast as I could, not bothering to look back to see if he was still with me.

WHEN I REACHED THE highway, having lost track of how long ago I'd left John behind, the air felt thick and humid. The road was mostly empty of cars, and the light was bright, giving the day a feeling of harshness. My mouth was dry. Distantly, I heard the sound of a siren as an ambulance approached.

My anger gave way to fear. *What if something happened to him? What if those were my last words to him?* I could not lose him; he was my rock. I began to cry, embarrassed and frustrated. I pulled my phone from my pocket to call him, but it went to voicemail. Was he not answering because something had happened or because the cell service was bad? I felt myself start to panic.

Just then, he rode up next to me. "I could tell you needed some space," he said.

"I thought something happened to you," I said, wiping my tears away. I sighed heavily. "I was so mad I couldn't see straight." We rode home in silence.

Back at the house, taking off his helmet, John looked at me. "Amy, I need to talk to you," he said. "I can't take all this on."

"What do you mean?" I said.

"I can't mount the cavalry for you," he said. "I can't be the middleman in all of this. It isn't good for either of us."

"I know," I said. "You're right. But I can't do this on my own, and I don't know where to go from here." I looked at him helplessly. John was always rational, skilled at solving problems. Why couldn't he solve this one?

Later, over video, I told Lauren about the bike ride, her sympathetic face nodding along on my iPad. "It just makes me feel so alone," I said. "I thought we were in this together."

"Amy," she said. "Have you thought about John's role in all of this? I think he just performed the most incredible act of love."

"What are you talking about?" I said. "It was devastating to hear that from him."

"He's your husband," she said. "He's not your investigator. He's not your lawyer. He's not your doctor. It's more than enough for one person to be sitting with you on the floor, holding your hand when you are crumbling. This man is in complete emotional service to you. Let that be enough."

She was right. I softened. It had been an act of care for him to set that boundary with me, to know that I needed a different kind of help from what he could provide. Just because it didn't feel good in the moment didn't mean that it wasn't important.

When I came downstairs, I found John with his cup of coffee in the kitchen. "John," I said, "I'm sorry." There was a long pause. "I needed a place to deposit my anger, and you're all I have."

"You don't need to apologize," he said. "I know how hard this is. It's new territory for all of us."

"Thank you," I said, taking a deep breath. I knew that he was on my side.

.   .   .

FEELING MORE RESOLVED, I tore into the report that had been sent to John. Much of it reiterated what Courtney had already found from Mr. Mason's social media, but assembled, it was a clearer picture of his biography.

The background check had primarily drawn upon court documents and other public records, but there was nothing out of the ordinary—only that the investigators hadn't been able to confirm that he attended the university he claimed on his social media. I wondered what else he'd lied about. But he had never been arrested; he wasn't a registered sex offender. He appeared to be like many of the men I knew back home in Texas: pro-gun, religiously affiliated, a lover of the outdoors. What he'd done to me was so horrifying it seemed unfathomable that there would be no trace of it in his record—although I knew that logically, there shouldn't be. What was I expecting from this report—a typed confession?

One detail haunted me, pulled from something he'd posted on social media a few years earlier: *He still drove the same car.* I thought back to the memory that had stuck with me, of seeing him pull away in the parking lot as I stood on the curb, after school, watching him.

I set the papers down, lying in bed next to John, and sighed. He looked over at me. "What are you thinking?"

Just then my phone lit up—a text from Courtney. I read it: "I just checked, and it looks like there's no statute of limitations on rape in the state of Texas."

I looked down at the papers, then back to John. I showed him Courtney's text.

"I think it's time we find you a good lawyer," John said. "Do you want me to make some inquiries, or is it something you want to do?"

"Thank you," I said. "I would love your help, as I'm not dealing well with the practical side of life right now. Again, I'm really sorry about the bike ride."

"It's okay," he said, and I knew that it was.

I thought about William's advice: It wasn't just about handling the external search for justice. The internal work was just as important, if not more. It had been a little over a month since my first session, which meant that I could safely do another one. "And I think I'm ready for my next session with Olivia," I said.

John nodded. "Are you going in for healing, or are you going to try to get more information?"

"Both," I said. I thought about Mr. Mason's car again. What else was there for me to remember that might connect the dots between the past and the present? Scrolling through social media, I'd seen a quote from Carl Jung that resonated: "Until we make the unconscious conscious, it will direct our life and we will call it fate." I was determined to unearth whatever I'd been ascribing to fate. "I want to put myself in control."

BOUNDARIES, I THOUGHT. THOSE were the key. I'd always had trouble with boundaries. I saw it most in my relationship to work, my willingness to stretch myself thin to fit in one more meeting or join one more conference call. I wore my busyness like a badge of honor. As work culture had gone more remote, I'd used it as an excuse to make myself even more available, wherever I was. Even now, mere weeks after the MDMA session that had upended my entire sense of self, I was in meetings, trying to stay focused while my mind wandered back to the middle-school bathroom. Likewise I had known in my efforts to be a supermom that I had been pushing myself past what was healthy—wanting to pretend for my kids that I was fine, when in reality I was reeling.

I thought about boundaries when an email popped up from James, with whom I had maintained a friendly relationship over the years, even socializing with his family now that he was married and was raising kids in Connecticut. He had written to ask me for recommendations, as he was planning an upcoming vacation. I quickly hit Reply to respond, as I always did. But then I paused. A part of me whispered: *Why are you still letting this man who raped you have a role in your life?*

Suddenly I felt embarrassed. How shameful, how pathetic, that I made space for a friendship with him. I imagined myself in a courtroom as a fictional defense attorney brought out my warm correspondence with James as exhibits on the stand, proof that I had been a willing participant in our relationship, that my claims were groundless because I'd been nice to him for so long. Not that I could imagine pursuing criminal charges against him; if anything, I tried scrupulously to keep him happy. I continued to go back to the well, imagining that it would make me feel better about myself to be closer to him, as if a positive relationship in the present would change the past.

I deleted his email without responding. *How's that for boundaries?* I thought.

The night before my second MDMA session with Olivia, I found myself thinking about all the ways men had talked about my body. I had been ten when I went to cotillion for the father-daughter dance and a boy sneered at me, "Nobody's ever going to want to dance with you because you have chicken legs." Or the Christmas after my first semester of college, when I'd come back to Amarillo. Walking into a family friend's house, I found some kids from high school, along with my high school boyfriend. A hush fell over the room as I entered. I had done the unthinkable by going to college so far from home, and here I was, back again. Somebody made a crack about my legs; I had gained the freshman fifteen, a mix of muscle and the bagels I ate for fuel as a stressed-out college athlete, and I couldn't remember exactly what was said, but I remembered the feeling—of shame and self-consciousness, which I stuffed down and tried to ignore as I always did.

All those ways in which I'd allowed men to take advantage of my polite compliance—that was over. I was done participating in a culture where men felt entitled to my body. That ex-boyfriend who had always wanted more from me in high school. The boys criticizing this body of mine that had endured so much for the apparent offense of getting stronger—how dare they? James, who raped me, then had the audacity to ask for a favor? How dare they all?

And yet it was John with whom I'd gotten so upset because his love made it safe for me to be angry. With all these other men, I couldn't allow myself the indulgence of my rage. I had cosigned their bad behavior with my southern gentility for too long.

Enough was enough.

FOR MY SECOND MDMA session, I felt no nerves. All I wanted was more information to be revealed, as it had been in the first. I lay down on the couch, secured the eyeshade, and dove in headfirst, with Olivia by my side.

After a few minutes, something began to swirl in my field of darkness. As I focused on the swirling, it became an arm, pulling me along the floor. It was him. Mr. Mason. We were back in the bathroom.

"It's the same thing as before," I said. "Only it's from a different angle. The first time, it was like I was watching from the corner of the room. Now I'm in it, seeing it through my own eyes."

I sat on the toilet, shirtless again. His hands were touching what little breasts I had as a twelve-year-old, grabbing at me as he jammed his penis in my mouth. I was choking. I could feel his pubic hair on my face.

"This time I feel the feelings," I said. "Last time I didn't feel anything." The emotions shot through me. "Panic. Terror. Sadness."

I watched as I fell off the toilet again against the wall. He grabbed me by the arm and dragged me onto the bathroom floor. Again there was new sensation, things I hadn't felt in my first session. The floor, cool and hard. I looked up at the handle of the door, longing to open it, to be anywhere but there.

I crawled to the wall and turned around to face him, sitting up against it, resting my back against the tile. I could feel my exhaustion and my fear. But I didn't show him that. Instead I smiled.

"I am smiling," I said to Olivia. "I am smiling because I'm hoping that if I do that, if I seem like I'm having a good time, it will be enough for him to set me free." *The same way I always did, the way I still do. Smiling to make a man comfortable.*

Instead I heard his voice, that Texas twang reverberating in my mind. "Have you had enough?" he asked. His boot pressed down on my lower back again.

In the session, I squirmed, as if I were trying to get away. "It just keeps repeating," I said to Olivia, "but I have seen all this before."

Then, in a flash, I was in a different memory. Now I was driving my car—the trusty blue Blazer with which my father had surprised me. "Thank God," I said. "Something besides the abuse. I'm older here." I was pulling up to the tennis center for what would be a match; I knew that because I was wearing a tennis skirt and a team shirt, with my hair pulled back in a ponytail.

As I parked, I looked through the windshield and saw him standing there. Mr. Mason. My hands shook. *No*, I thought.

"No," I said out loud, back in the session. "No, no."

In the memory, I fumbled with my keys, attached to a Dooney & Bourke leather keychain, which had a ring of plastic frames attached to it. I had filled the frames with photographs of my best friends. I looked down at their faces, pretending to be distracted by the pictures. When I raised my head to look back up at Mr. Mason, he was smiling and waving at me.

I got out of the car and walked over to him, standing on the sidewalk.

"One more time," he said, "for old times' sake?"

I nodded, and numbly I followed him into the tennis team room.

YOU'D ASSUME THAT REMEMBERING this, I'd have thought, *But wasn't I sixteen then?* I must have wondered, *Why didn't I stop him?* I must have thought, *How could he have done this in such a public place? Why didn't I say no?* I must have thought, *Where were my boundaries?*

But I didn't think any of that. Held in the golden arms of the medicine, the compassion I felt for young Amy was absolute.

Of course he had power over me; he was the keeper of my greatest shame. Of course I did what he wanted me to do; I was terrified of him, and even more terrified of the secret. This was where I learned how to keep myself safe, how to survive. Those were the only boundaries I knew.

6. SIGNS

The lawyer arrived at my house promptly at ten. Her name was Cate, and she was a trim woman with a sleek brown bob, dressed perfectly in shades of blanched khaki and cream.

"Sorry I'm dressed so casually," she said. "It's the weekend." I caught my reflection in the mirror: workout pants, white sunscreen smeared across my face, and my hair matted from the baseball cap I'd been wearing. The days of trying to pull it together, for me, were now a distant memory.

My enormous oaf of a dog slobbered over her pant leg as she entered the house. "Hey!" I yelled. "Knock it off!" I pushed his nose away. "I'm so sorry," I said to her. "He's just looking for attention."

Like the company that had prepared the initial report on

my abuser, Cate had been recommended to me by a business contact. Her approach was purposeful and direct, yet there was a softness to her that made me feel that I could trust her.

I had gotten better at telling my story. These admissions continued to feel both like a profound act of catharsis and like their own trauma: It was something I knew I had to do but the act of recounting would frequently knock me out for the rest of the day. I'd begun to understand that the more I repeated it, the less shame I would feel, and so it was important to articulate, but that didn't make it any easier.

As I told Cate my story, she popped in with occasional questions. "What is MMD . . . ?" she asked at one point, trailing off. I was self-conscious trying to explain to this poised, polished woman that I had retrieved these memories through use of an illegal substance. Talking with her, I felt like her skepticism was merited. "I'll read up on it," she said reassuringly.

"The memories didn't all come through when I was on the drug," I said, a little defensively. "I think the drug just gave me permission to open the door."

She nodded. "So, from a legal perspective, what is your desired outcome?" she asked.

"I don't know yet," I said. "I want to do what's right."

"I understand," she said. "In most of these cases, it's about money. So let's play this out. You're wealthier than your former teacher. If you bring charges, there's a chance he'll come after you for defamation."

"There's no other option," I said. "I need to validate my memories. He can't get away with this. What if he's still hurting people?"

"Is there anything that would deter you from wanting to take legal action against him?"

I thought about it. "Only if it would somehow harm my children," I said. The most important thing in the world was keeping my kids safe—from real threats, not the things that I'd cared about before. What difference did it make if my kids were parading around the house with a box of cookies minutes before dinner? What mattered was that I find some way to protect them, both from the world and from what this might to do to them. Was I bringing my trauma too close to them? Would it affect their lives adversely? In my refusal to acknowledge my pain, what if I had blocked my ability to see theirs?

As a parent, you could only stay on top of things that fell within your purview. I'd spent so much time ensuring there were plastic plugs covering every electrical outlet and diving to cover corners of tables when one of my kids was sure to hit their head—but those things were concrete, external. How could I protect my children from threats I couldn't see?

"I think your children will have so much respect for you when you tell them your story," she said. I hoped she was right, but the thought of telling my children now was daunting. I wasn't sure I could bear telling them this. Would it damage them to learn something so difficult about their mother? I wasn't even sure what emotion I wanted them to feel. Did I want them to be sad for me? I knew that I didn't want them to have to parent me.

"So what can I expect from this process?" I asked. "I don't know anything about how the law works."

"Well, with the little bit of research I've done, it appears that the statute of limitations has passed for criminal cases," she said. "But that doesn't mean we can't pursue a civil case."

"I thought there was no statute of limitations on rape cases in Texas," I said, remembering what Courtney had told me.

Cate's brow furrowed. "Let me check on that."

"Obviously, I have no physical evidence," I said. As I thought about it, a flashback sliced through my memory. I was back in the bathroom with him, using my kneepads from volleyball to wipe up his bodily fluid. I closed my eyes, then opened them, looking back at Cate. "Also," I said, "it's been thirty years. I don't even know yet if there are other victims." I shifted in my seat. "Let me rephrase that. I know there are probably other victims, but I don't know how we'd go about finding them or if they'd come forward. It's been such a long time, and people don't want to dive into the past. For now, I have to operate under the assumption that I'm the only survivor."

"We can have an investigator start making some calls," Cate said.

"Let's just be as discreet as possible about that," I said. "I am still keeping this a secret from my family. I'm not sure when I'm going to tell them."

"Understood," Cate said. "Can you start thinking about who we should be talking to?"

"Bess Taylor," I said. "She was my coach. I knew she cared about me. She could have some answers."

Cate nodded. "Who else?"

"The other person," I said, "is a girl named Claudia. My friend already found her online. She was a classmate of mine at the school. I believe she knows something."

"Why do you say that?"

"I have several distinct memories of the two of them together," I said. I felt like my throat was closing up. I was suddenly nauseous. "Maybe it was happening to her, too."

"We'll start on the periphery and then move in closer to

avoid tipping him off," she said. "I know it's a small town." Then she studied me. "Are you all right?" she asked.

I nodded, but the truth was, I felt sick.

"I'm so sorry," Cate said. "I have kids too, you know." Then she steeled herself. "We've got to get this guy. But we've got to get our ducks in a row before we go after him. There's a process to all of this."

I nodded. "I'm ready. Let's do it."

THAT WEEKEND, JOHN PLANNED a getaway for us back down south, to a farm we'd visited years before. It was one of my most beloved places: We would go for bike rides up and down lush green hills, pedaling under covered bridges alongside a meandering river.

This part of the country had once been sacred to me, but now there were new triggers. Riding past a wheat field, I noticed a sign that marked it as property of the university where Mason had gone to school, or rather, where he'd claimed he'd gone to school, since the background check hadn't been able to prove his attendance. The sight of it soured my mood.

That evening, I couldn't stop thinking about the sign as I drifted off to sleep. How hadn't anyone uncovered what a liar he was? How was he even hired in the first place? And how did he get away with it? Why wasn't anyone paying attention? I was furious with everyone: parents, teachers, coaches, this so-called community that claimed to put family first. And most of all, I was furious with myself, for having hidden it for so long.

In the night, I awakened to the image of a face. In my mind, clear as a picture, was Bess Taylor, my eighth-grade volleyball coach, the one who had given me the award in the auditorium. I had always thought fondly of her; every so often my mother would mention to me that she'd run into her. "Coach Taylor asked all about you and what you were up to," she'd say. "You know she's not teaching anymore? She's been working at a juice bar in town." Even years later, if I'd been asked who had influenced me the most in my years as a student athlete, I would have cited Bess as the coach who believed in me most fiercely and gave me my start.

"Everyone, look at Amy!" she had called. I had always remembered that; I could hear her voice in my memory. It was no wonder: The second I walked through the locker-room door, I was in practice mode. I'd throw on my volleyball clothes, grab the jump rope for a warm-up, and keep jumping in the corner for as long as I could, never taking a breath, never chatting with friends—the other girls around me, who were joking and tripping over their ropes. That wasn't me. I was focused and ready. I would not miss a turn of the rope—locked and loaded, refusing to take my eye off the ball. Decades later, I could still feel the surging intensity rippling through my body, knowing I needed to work harder than everyone else.

Why was I so rigid? I saw Bess's expectant face in my mind's eye—the way she always praised me, how she'd tell the other girls to work as hard as I did. She, too, saw me the way I wanted to be seen. *Did I always practice so intensely because I thought I could hide behind that focus?*

And then I was back in the auditorium again, watching Bess cry as she introduced me. There was no memory more vivid in my mind than this one. But I had always focused my attention on my own feelings in that moment—the curiosity

I'd felt about this extraordinary girl Bess was describing; the jolt when I learned it was me; the expressions on my parents' faces, my father's tears. I had always been so grateful to Bess for seeing my full potential, for believing in me and acknowledging my hard work.

But now, for the first time, I was curious about her tears. *Why was she crying so hard?*

I could see now that Bess was always overwhelmed. She was constantly running her hands through her hair, fidgeting anxiously. I was particularly compliant with her because I could tell how flustered she would get when the other girls didn't follow the rules, and I wanted to spare her the discomfort of having to be a disciplinarian, since it clearly wasn't her temperament. I had tried to help her. I was angry, now, that she hadn't been able to help me—that no adults had been able to help me. I had wondered many times over the last two months how I ended up in so many of the spaces where the abuse happened without anyone noticing. Where were the adults who were supposed to be protecting me? Why were they so distracted?

I would find Mr. Mason chatting with Coach Taylor right before practice. He would stand outside the locker-room door, laughing with her, rocking back and forth on his cowboy boots as I passed them to go change my clothes. Maybe they were friends; maybe she liked his attention. Maybe it was her own insecurities that prevented her from seeing what was right in front of her.

If only she had known that Mason was waiting for me under the bleachers, where he'd told me to meet him. He raped me there, too. I could hear his voice. "Get up," he said. "Hurry, so no one sees us." Where were all the grown-ups?

"Amy?" I heard John's voice.

"Some stuff is coming through for me," I said.

"Do you want me to turn the light on?" He switched on a lamp, and I saw his kind, concerned face. "What can I do to help?"

"Can you just put your hand on my back?" I said. I took deep breaths. "If we're going to ride tomorrow, I've got to get some sleep." I felt furious and confused—how was I supposed to trust anyone when I felt so betrayed by those I had trusted?

RACHEL AND COURTNEY CHECKED in on me frequently; I suspected they were coordinating behind the scenes to make sure that I wasn't going off the rails, but I accepted that kindness. When I was spiraling, a friendly text centered me. But it was a delicate dance: I could tell they were trying to figure out how best to help me, and yet I rarely knew what I needed—other than to keep untangling my memories.

In my next session with Lauren, I tried to process the fact that a coach whom I had loved so much had failed to recognize what was happening to me. "I liked Bess," I said. "I trusted her. And even more importantly, she believed in me. Why couldn't she see that I was suffering?"

"How much do you remember about that time in her life?"

"Not much," I said. "I was a child. She was an authority figure to me." I shook my head. "If there's anyone I can talk to about this, it's her."

"Let's slow down and be curious about it," Lauren said. "Of course, if you want to talk to her, that's your choice. But let's be sure your decision comes from a place of consideration and care, not impulsiveness. Pay attention to what's happening to your nervous system. Talking about the investigation seems to get you activated."

Lauren wasn't wrong. When Cate and I met again to discuss how the investigation was moving along, I was surprised to learn how much research had already been conducted. Among my fellow classmates from Navarro, there seemed to be two camps: those who remembered Mason fondly and those who characterized him as being ambiently creepy, known for giving female students rides off campus in his car, which would certainly have been verboten. I could picture his car in my mind's eye, but I couldn't remember whether he'd ever given me a ride; it was just that one image that had endured, of him pulling out of the faculty parking lot in his car after school, just the two of us— me standing on the curb, watching him drive away. The investigator hadn't reached out to Coach Taylor yet.

I scanned the files as Cate summarized the highlights for me. "One girl said a friend of hers woke up during an overnight school trip to find him standing in the room, watching the girls sleeping, and it frightened her," she said. "That was the extent of it. Nothing more than that happened."

"But that was secondhand?" I said. "She didn't see it herself? What about the girl who actually saw it?"

"Allie," Cate said, checking her notes. "She left town, apparently, and nobody's heard from her in years. The investigator tried to get her contact information, but it sounds like people don't want to get involved."

"Everybody's got skeletons in a small town," I said.

"I'm sorry we don't have much more in the way of answers for you."

"And how about Claudia?" I asked. I thought back to that

image I'd had of her: Mr. Mason's hand on her shoulder. The way she looked returning my dress that day, standing on my doorstep while I hid in my bedroom.

"Oh, yes," Cate said smoothly. "We got in touch with her. I'm afraid she didn't remember much."

"What do you mean?"

"She had no recollections of Mason, or any other salient memories of those years at the school. She barely remembered you." Cate looked up at me. "Were you close?"

"No," I said. "Not close. I just thought . . ." I felt defeated. "I don't know what I thought."

"And what about your coach—what's her name?"

"Bess," I said. "Bess Taylor. I think I'm going to call her myself." I turned the folder of documents over. On the front, it was labeled: CONFIDENTIAL: PROJECT LONGHORN.

Cate looked mildly abashed.

"We've been calling it Project Longhorn for privacy purposes," she said. "Since you're from Texas and all." *From Texas,* I thought. For a moment I longed to be back there, in the garage of my parents' house, helping my mom make homemade mint ice cream—crushing bags of hard peppermint candies, the sound of the silver canister crunching against layers of ice and rock salt for hours until it was finally ready, creamy and cold and bright pink. Now the sweetness of the memory pained me. Would I ever want to go home again?

SUMMER HAD ENDED, AND my kids were back in school. Walking with Gigi and Gracie to drop them off a few blocks from our apartment, I found myself thinking about all the people who had been around when my own abuse had gone on. Was it really possible that something so heinous could have been happening and that none of the faculty could have known? How scary a thought that we entrust our children to the care of others, not knowing exactly what might be going on when they are out of our sight for so many hours. I knew that my girls were in the best hands, and they were so busy with friends and scheduled activities. Still, the fear plagued me: My children were so vulnerable, as I had been.

As we arrived at the school, the girls chatting amiably and checking their phones one last time before the school day began, I saw their favorite teacher, Clara, standing in the lobby. She was an elegant woman with long, dark hair and kind eyes, whom I'd come to consider a close friend. As my daughters bounded up the stairs, she once-overed me.

"Are you doing all right, Amy?" she said kindly.

"I'm fine," I said wearily. "Just a lot on my plate."

She nodded briskly. She had too much decorum to push. "You know I'm always here."

I looked at this kind, intelligent woman and knew she'd never let anyone, anything, harm my daughters. Still, I couldn't shake the fear I felt in my body. I had to do more to keep my kids safe. That night, I checked in with Julian.

"Mom, I'm so annoyed," he said. "I traded something in a video game, and the other player never transferred the coin he was supposed to send me." He looked perturbed. "I trusted him!"

This was a perfect opening for me. "How do you know when someone is trustworthy?" I asked. "Have you played with this other person before?"

"No," he said.

"Well, people need to earn our trust. But sometimes these mistakes help us learn things, because not everyone who earns our trust deserves to keep it." I didn't want to scare my eight-year-old. Maybe I had gone too far.

"I know, Mom," he said. "But I gotta get that coin back. It makes me so mad."

I ran my hand over the top of his head. "You have every right to be upset," I said. "The important thing is that you learn to lean on your instincts."

FROM THE MOMENT I recovered memories of what happened, I had taken copious notes—documenting everything I was feeling, keeping journals of exactly what I was doing as I moved through this surreal new life where I was, suddenly, leading an investigation into my own decades-old assault. On calls, I scribbled down details on napkins and in the margins of books, trying to keep track of how everything was unfolding. So many of my old priorities—from the opinions of other moms on the playground to the endless hours I'd once spent exercising—now felt frivolous. Who gave a shit about the font of our Christmas card when all I could think about was the way the tile of that bathroom wall felt against my forehead? What mattered now was that I find Mason, corroborate my experience, and make sure he could never hurt anyone else ever again.

I had mostly stopped second-guessing that the abuse had happened; I knew, as sturdily as I had felt in my first MDMA session, that it had. The memories could not have been more concrete. And yet I needed something solid, external, *outside* of my own memory to back me up so other people would believe me. Wasn't that how it worked in a court of law? I needed evidence, not just the shockingly vivid image of a toilet paper holder that I grabbed on to as I was dragged to the floor—a memory that had endured after thirty years but one that didn't prove anything to anyone but me.

I was growing more anxious. What if I forgot a detail that I'd recalled in my sessions? What if I left something out when talking to someone that might lead to a clue that substantiated what I'd remembered? What if, as much as my insights would fuse together days after an MDMA session, I failed to realize how important some detail was in the moment? I couldn't write everything down fast enough. I was having a hard time remembering anything happening in the real world; I slept poorly and felt spacey. I'd hidden something so huge from my conscious mind for decades, it was difficult for me to trust my own discernment.

Maybe this was why, without giving it much thought, I began recording my sessions with Lauren. Recording our conversations made them feel real, sturdy, tangible. It felt like a form of self-care. There could be no take-backs, because I knew I had it on the record—even if it was for nobody else but me to ever hear. It wasn't even about listening to it later—I just needed to know that there was a record of my experience, something credible to substantiate what I had been thinking or feeling at the time. When my own past had been lost to me for so many years, I wanted to make the present as solid as I could—and recording felt like the way to do that.

Through the small-town grapevine, I was able to obtain Bess's number. "I have been meaning to reach out to you for years," I texted her. "You always believed in me and gave me my start in volleyball." She responded immediately. "I would love to talk to you!" she wrote. "I tell everyone you were always my favorite kid." Then: "One more thing, Amy. Your mom's Christmas card is the highlight of my Christmas every year. I love watching your entire family grow!" I wasn't sure whether to feel like I was being disingenuous. I wasn't calling to catch up with her; I was curious to see what I could find out. I remembered the feeling of how much Bess had cared about me. It felt good to reconnect with the person who'd once made me feel that way. But as soon as I thought that, I remembered that I'd thought Mason cared about me too. Once again I was left perplexed, unable to trust my own understanding of other people. Bess and I made a plan to speak by phone that weekend.

Her voice was exactly the same: a kindly southern drawl with a touch of static that hinted at a tough past. We caught up for nearly an hour, talking about career, kids, and shared connections back in Amarillo—though we'd both long since moved away. "You know, I followed in your footsteps and helped coach the varsity team at my daughter's school for two seasons," I told her.

"I'm sure in thirty years' time, you'll hear from those girls about what a difference you made in their lives," she laughed. I told her that I was still close with Courtney and Rachel, and she remembered them both vividly. "Rachel was such a little powerhouse," she said fondly. "And Courtney was so determined—willing to do whatever it took. Do you remember when I gave you that award?"

"I was so confused when you said my name," I said. "Why was I getting an award for being kind? Weren't we always supposed to be kind?"

"Well, you were always special to me, Amy," she said. Then she sounded briefly irked. "I wish I could look through my yearbooks now, but I sent them to Mr. Mason when all that junk started with him. You heard about all that, right?"

My palms began to sweat. "What junk with Mr. Mason?" I said. I held my breath.

"Oh, there were folks calling around asking questions about him—somebody making some allegations against him," she said. I suspected that was Cate's team. "So I picked up the phone and warned him about it! Hadn't talked to him in decades, but I had to tell him what I was hearing. Nothing's come of it, so maybe they backed off. Seems like the whole thing was bogus. That man was amazing."

I made a noise that sounded like I was both surprised and distressed to learn this. "He must have been sad about that," I said.

"Oh, he was heartbroken!" Bess said. "I don't know if you remember him."

"Yes." I took a breath. "I ran for student council president and lost. He told me that I was the real leader of the school."

She must have heard the edge in my voice, because when she spoke again, her voice cracked.

"Amy, did you have a problem with him?"

I was silent.

"Amy?"

The quiet between us was unbearable.

"Oh my gosh, Amy," she said. "If you had a problem with him and I stood up for him, I need to know."

I let the silence on the line speak volumes, knowing it could say what I couldn't. "I think I know what happened," she said. I could hear tears in her voice, and the sound of them made me begin to cry too. "My heart is breaking for you. Amy, you have to know—the only reason I called him was because I heard there were allegations against him and I didn't believe it. But I didn't know it was you. I'll never talk to him again. I promise. I was wrong to support him."

"Bess—" I said.

"I'm calling him to get my yearbooks back," she said.

"Don't!" I said. "Please don't do that."

I took a deep breath. Finally, my voice shaking, I told her my story. Every detail. She was silent as I spoke, but I could feel through the phone that it hit her hard.

"I don't know how I didn't see it, Amy," Bess said. "Honestly, I don't. I owe you an apology for missing it." She choked back a sob. She sounded genuinely anguished. How could she possibly have known? And yet just a few days earlier, waking up in that hotel room, I had felt so angry and alone. "I was abused myself as a girl, and I just hit the ground running as soon as I graduated. I was so young, Amy. I don't know if you realized that, but I was only twenty-one when I started coaching you. And I was responsible for over three hundred kids a day. There were days I just couldn't cope, and there was so little support at the school. I don't want to sound like I'm making excuses. It was just a hard time."

Listening to Bess, I saw her now as the overwhelmed young adult she'd been. I had called her hoping that she would corroborate my every memory. But I myself had been incapable of seeing the truth for so long; surely I had to extend her the same benefit of the doubt. She cared so much about me—and was so friendly with him—if anyone could have seen what was happening, it would have been her. And yet I hadn't even known myself. Isn't that what I had done all the years I had run from my past? Isn't that what happens when you've been abused—that you can't see what is right in front of you?

All those years, the memories lurked below the surface of conscious thought, inaccessible to me, until finally they bubbled up. Consider how I had maintained my own cozy relationship with James, even though I knew exactly what he'd done to me.

Abuse, I was beginning to understand, was a tangled mess of shame and silence. The abused learn early that survival sometimes means protecting the secrets of their abusers. Growing up doesn't mean that impulse goes away. I had reached out to Bess hoping that she would remember something that would confirm my experience, but she didn't have any revelations that could help me to begin to understand things more clearly or bring Mr. Mason to justice.

So instead, I listened. I listened as she told me about the abuse in her childhood that she'd blotted out and then come to terms with, and about the closure she was still chasing. She kept apologizing for having missed what was happening to me, but I wasn't angry with her anymore. I knew all too well how it was easier not to see.

By the time we hung up the phone, I realized Bess and I had more in common than I'd thought. We both had teenage boys who loved to fish and girls who played volleyball. We had both survived the unthinkable.

Talking to Bess that night, I hoped that her kids were safe, that she had found peace.

I hoped someday she'd get her yearbooks back.

7. SECRETS

L ife had never slowed down, but as I'd continued to sort through what I'd uncovered, John had stepped in, making sure the kids got their booster shots and braces tightened. The straightness of my kids' teeth couldn't have been further from my mind. How could I proceed with parent-teacher conferences and lunches with colleagues when I was plagued by persistent flashbacks—memories that reminded me that this was still unresolved, that Mr. Mason was still out there, and that I had done nothing to bring him to justice? Lauren kept telling me that I needed to focus on myself, but I didn't know how to do that—I felt that the thing I needed most, what would feel like the deepest self-care, would be for my memories to be corroborated.

"I have to gather as many facts as I can," I insisted to my

computer screen, where Lauren was on video, seated in her office. "Don't you see? Me getting hard facts proves that this all really happened. That it's not all in my head." As much as I trusted my own memories, I felt insecure that nothing in the physical world had confirmed that they were real—that we hadn't found any other survivors, that nobody who knew me then had seen the signs. I knew that the people in my inner circle with whom I'd shared my story believed me, but would anyone else? "It would make it so much easier to tell my parents if I could prove it somehow," I said.

"That's an interesting thought," Lauren said. "As though your word isn't enough, even for the people who love you. Like you still need to prove something to them—and maybe to yourself."

"It's about holding him accountable—that's how I will heal," I said. "Justice is how I heal, for me and for everyone else who's been through something like this. What kind of example am I setting for my daughters, and for other women, if I don't do everything I can to make sure he can't hurt anyone else?"

"That sounds like something really important to explore," Lauren said patiently. "What would justice look like to you?"

"Well, I don't know," I said. "Cate's the one who's working on the legal strategy. That's her job."

When I met with Cate at my office, she had energizing news. "Your friend was right. There is no longer a statute of limitations on rape cases in the state of Texas," she said.

"Really?" I said, but I wasn't surprised. Courtney was never wrong.

"It's confusing because they've changed the laws over the years," she said. "But if you so choose, you can bring forth criminal charges. You'll have to spend a lot of time in a Texas courthouse, but if this is what you want, we can absolutely pursue it. The other option is to pursue a civil case, but I worry in that instance he'll countersue, and you could be looking at a very long and arduous legal battle that leads to nowhere."

"My friend William was able to bring charges against his abuser," I said. "The system worked in his favor. Why wouldn't it work in mine?"

"Well," Cate said, "there were multiple victims in that case, weren't there?"

"Yes," I said. "The school sent a letter to former students and several others came forward. That's why I'm hoping there's someone else who will come forward about Mr. Mason." I hesitated. "There's also a part of me that's afraid nobody else will come forward. After all, it was such a long time ago, in such a conservative place. And then there's also a part of me that just hopes it didn't happen to anyone else."

The possibility of pursuing a criminal case felt like a step forward. Pursuing criminal charges was a tangible, external thing I could do in the real world.

"So what are our next steps?" I asked.

"Well, I don't know that a corporate New York lawyer is the right person to start banging down the sheriff's door in West Texas," Cate said. "It might be better if you had someone on the ground who can help you navigate the landscape. And it should probably be a man."

"My dad knows everyone in Amarillo," I said.

"What about confidentiality?"

"Tough to keep people from talking in a small town," I said, sighing. "I think I'm at the point where I need to tell my family. I'm going to see my sister."

. . .

AFTER COLLEGE, LIZZIE HAD settled in Fort Worth with her husband, Rob, with whom she had five children. Though we were close, we were very different. Lizzie had inherited my mother's abilities as a caretaker; she was a supermom, endlessly patient and nurturing, a wiz with her mother-in-law's pancake recipe and juggling the responsibilities of raising five kids in rapid succession with little outside help. I had inherited more of my father's leadership style and powers of delegation; I could barely tell a microwave from a stove. The most time I ever spent in my kitchen was making a binder of takeout menus. I hid anything I confiscated from my kids, like candy or iPads, in the oven, because I knew it was the one place no one would ever look. I envied Lizzie when I'd see her in her robe and slippers, the same style my mom wore when she clomped up and down the hall in the morning to wake us up for school. Lizzie was comfortable in a domestic life that had never come as easily to me. I loved her deeply, but I also sensed that she wanted more from our relationship, something I never knew how to give.

When I told her I was coming to see her, I could hear the excitement in her voice. "Of course I'll make the time!" she said. "I can get someone to help me with the kids!"

"Hey, don't mention that I'm coming to Mom," I said. "You know she'll jump on a plane and come visit us, and you and I never get to spend time together. We don't want to hurt her feelings." I had decided that I needed to tell Lizzie first, to be certain that nothing like this had happened to her too. I knew that it would devastate me if I told my parents and my mother's first question was *What about Lizzie—did she have him as a teacher?* It was critical that I have an answer prepared, that I be able to reassure her that Lizzie hadn't been abused too.

"I'm so excited to see you," Lizzie said. "Let me know what you're thinking."

"Well, I have a meeting in Dallas, but I'll stay an extra day," I said. "Why don't you come stay at the hotel with me? We can spend the day together and really catch up."

"That sounds great," Lizzie said, beaming. "Thank you so much for making time for me."

My hands shook as I checked into the hotel with her standing behind me, filling me in on her latest project at work and updates on the kids. I couldn't even pretend to listen. I felt like I was on a mission. I just had to tell her.

"I made us a reservation at my favorite little spot in town," she was saying. "Or we could do some shopping—what sounds fun to you?" I looked at her. "I'm just so happy to be together."

"Let's go up to the room and get settled," I said. I was trying to sound casual if only to keep myself calm, but I felt like I was lying to her.

Trudging down that hallway was the longest walk of my life. She was exuberant, and I was about to crush her. The minute the heavy hotel room door swung closed, before I'd even turned on the lights, I took a deep breath and spoke. "Lizzie," I said, "the real reason I came here is because I have to tell you something."

She looked confused. "What?"

"I have to tell you about some things that happened when we were growing up," I said. "We should sit down."

As I talked, her eyes began to look glassy. Her chin dropped. "What?" she said. "How is this possible? How did nobody see? And how are you just remembering this now?"

"I don't know," I said.

"Why didn't you tell anyone? Not even Courtney or Rachel?"

"Because I wasn't even honest with myself about it until just recently," I said. "I couldn't even tell myself the truth."

"But how did you come home after this had happened to you at school without anyone realizing?" she said. "Did you have bruises? Was there blood in your underwear?"

"I don't have answers to those questions," I said. Then, in a flash, I remembered the wedding video—how embarrassed I'd been by the footage of our babysitter talking about my stained underwear and how furious I had been with Lizzie for having included that detail. All this time, neither of us had understood why I'd been so hurt. Now it made sense.

"I knew there was another reason you were coming," Lizzie said. "You've never dropped in for no reason in the middle of a week. I told my best friend I was nervous about your visit. She said, 'Lizzie, you have nothing to be nervous about. She's your sister. She loves you. She might look good on paper, but you have so much more to offer her emotionally than she does you.'"

Hearing this blindsided me. I understood I had chosen a very different life from my siblings, having chased big dreams and followed my ambition out of Texas and to New York. I had never thought to wonder why. But I was starting to realize that moving so quickly was how I'd avoided acknowledging what had happened to me. How *could* I have much to offer my sister emotionally if I was always on the run? For that matter, had I been emotionally available for anyone? I had always prioritized achievement, focusing on the way things looked from the outside and how people saw me. I'd never slowed down enough to think about how things felt.

"Wow, that hurts," I said, taking it in. "Unfortunately, I think you might be right. But I need you now. In fact, I've never needed you more." I was stoic, composed. Ready to ask the heaviest question. "Lizzie, please tell me nothing happened to you."

"No!" she said emphatically. "I didn't even go to that school. I needed extra reading help, remember? I stayed in private school until ninth grade."

I exhaled a heavy sigh of relief. "Oh, that's right. Thank God."

Lizzie's phone had been vibrating next to her on and off for the last hour; she had been checking it but ignoring the calls. "Who is it?" I finally asked.

"It's Mom," she said.

"Do you need to answer?"

"Well, I told her how excited I was that you were coming. I just couldn't help myself—"

I pressed my hands to my temples. "Lizzie, I asked you not to tell her I was coming. I haven't figured out how to tell her what happened, and I don't know when I'm going to, and part of me telling you was figuring out how I'm going to do that—"

"I'm sorry—"

"We have to answer now," I said. Lizzie picked up the call.

"Hi, Mom!" she said, feigning as much excitement as she could muster.

My mother's voice, warm and sweet, crackled through the phone. "Are you there with Amy?"

"I'm here!" I said, trying to sound bright. "Hi, Mom! I

was just stopping through town, so I wanted to see Lizzie while I'm here!"

"Nothing makes me happier than knowing my two girls are together," she said. "I sure do wish I was there with you. Are you having fun?"

"Uh-huh," I said.

Lizzie and I stared at each other, crouched around the phone. In that moment, strange as it was, I felt a new kinship with her—a different type of connection. She knew my secret now. A wall that had stood between us forever had been torn down. Annoyed as I was that once again I had to pretend everything was fine, in this shared project, my sister and I had found each other.

We stayed in the room all day and night, ordering Domino's pizza at midnight. When I woke up the next morning, I could hear her sobbing in the bed next to me.

"I sometimes wondered why you were so sad," she said. "So sad but so driven. Like you were always on a mission. Trying to prove something. But I thought that's just how you were."

"Of course I was sad, Lizzie," I said. "Think about what was happening to me. I was so jealous of you because you seemed so free. I yearned to be that free. To have that abandon."

"I had no idea, Amy," she said. "I idolized you. All I wanted was for you to see me."

I felt torn. I wanted to make her feel better, but also, couldn't she be the one to make *me* feel better instead of the other way around? In that moment, I wished that the birth order had been reversed; I was the one who needed a big sister now. Wasn't I the one who had revealed a decades-old trauma? How was it possible that we'd both been hurting for so long, and neither of us ever spoke about it? Maybe we hadn't even realized it until now. "Lizzie, I do see you," I promised. "But I have been running so fast for so long that maybe there were things I never fully allowed myself to see." I took a breath. "Coming here to tell you this was one of the most difficult things I've ever had to do. The conversation with Mom and Dad will probably be the hardest day of my life. But I had to tell you first. I had to make sure you were okay."

She blew her nose. "Who else knows?"

"Courtney and Rachel," I said. She shook her head. "I knew how painful it would be for you to keep this from Mom," I said. "I didn't want to put you in that position."

She looked at me with swollen eyes. "When are you going to tell them?"

"Soon."

"This is going to kill them," she said. "Family is everything to them."

I nodded.

"How are you going to tell them?"

I sighed. "I don't know yet."

BACK IN NEW YORK, I felt like the days were blurring together. John brought me coffee each morning. I spent a lot of time in the bathtub. I stared numbly into the screen on video calls, letting my team at work carry the load. Shuffling down Madison Avenue, I ran into an old friend who did a double take when she saw me—unkempt, my eyes lowered to the ground, a shell of my old self. "I'm not in a good place,"

I said by way of explanation. I could barely bring myself to
hug her.

The only thing that brought me a familiar sense of joy
was being with my family—reading to Julian at night, cheer-
ing from the sidelines of my older kids' athletic events. My
children were focusing on their everyday triumphs and challenges. To be there for them, as I always had been, allowed
me a sense of normalcy.

Yet I was lost. Some days I walked through Central Park
for hours, aimlessly, looking up to find that I'd wandered
into a corner of the park that I barely recognized. But how
could I recognize where I was when I had come to barely
recognize myself?

"I don't know how I'm supposed to get back to normal
life," I said to Olivia. "I don't know how I'm going to drop
back into a normal life of dinner parties and small talk."

"Oh, Amy," she said softly. "You might not want to go to
those dinner parties anymore."

"I feel like I'm sinking deeper," I told Lauren during our
phone session. I was in the bathroom, perched on the edge
of the stone tub. "Sitting in that dark hotel room with my
sister, confronting everything I've been through. This is getting harder, not easier."

"What do you think you might need right now?" she
asked.

"The clearest need I have in this moment is for information," I said. "Memories. Concrete facts. Evidence. Something
I can hold on to. I'm scared it's going to go back in my brain
and disappear. That's why I've been—" I paused. It hit me out
of nowhere—a feeling of profound shame. "Lauren," I said, "I
forgot to tell you something. I've recorded our last two calls."

There was a long silence. "I find that interesting," she said. Her tone had changed. I felt like a child who had misbehaved. It seemed like she was upset, or maybe it was just that I was; I couldn't tell.

"I feel safe knowing that I have these conversations," I said. "I'm so out of it these days. I just—I want to be able to look back and know that this period of my life was real. Before, important things happened to me, and I forgot about them. I feel like I need to record everything now." I knew I was trying to justify my actions, trying to defend myself. "I just—I don't know how to move forward," I said.

"Well, it's interesting," Lauren said again.

"I didn't even think about the fact that there were two people involved," I said. "I'm so sorry. At first I was taking notes, and then I realized it would be easier to just record the conversation."

"Yes, but just like your past, Amy, this has to do with consent," she said.

"Consent?" I said. I could feel heat rising within me. "Are you implying that I'm victimizing you the same way I was victimized?"

"Were you recording us when we were together in person?"

"No!" I said. "Of course not!"

"Then can you help me understand why you feel the need to record me when I'm on the phone?"

"I've only done it once or twice," I protested. "I didn't even think about it." I started to cry.

"Amy, I'm not angry," she said. I couldn't compose myself. My whole body was trembling. Our time had ended, and I knew she had another call. "I give you my consent to record our conversations," she said. "But I would like to ask to be able to take it back at any time."

I yanked a robe off a hook and wrapped it around my face like a security blanket. "I'm so sorry," I said. "I think this is a bump we're going to have to get over."

"We will," she said. "I'm not going anywhere."

I believed her, but after the call ended, I sat trying to understand why I had reacted so strongly. How had my shame turned to defensiveness so quickly? I had acted like an embarrassed child. How could I not have considered her need for consent, especially given how loaded the subject was for me? Where was the disconnect?

Or had I been so defensive because I felt that I'd been shamed by an authority figure? I thought about what Lauren had said. She'd assured me that she wasn't angry; then we talked about boundaries. As much as it stung to be called out, I knew this was the mature way to build a real relationship.

Before my next session with Lauren, I checked in with Cate. She was constantly weighing the risks and rewards of whom we spoke to and how it might impact the outcome of the case. But her team was calling so many people in the community that my parents were bound to find out eventually. "I think we're at a point now, Amy, where anything we do might reach your parents," Cate said. I knew I couldn't wait any longer.

When I spoke to Lauren, she reassured me that our relationship hadn't been harmed. "I really wasn't mad at you," she said. "It's all part of what you're trudging through, in terms of how you feel safe and what makes you feel in control. But I think it's something for us to pay attention to, this question of where you are in your trust—in yourself and your story, and in me and our relationship." With her help, I tried to plot out the best way to have this unbearable conversation with my parents, even though I knew there was no way to prepare for something like this. I wrote bullet points, practicing how I would start off. I thought through how to deliver the news in a way that would stress key takeaways. I wanted to get this right. Even with this, I was still an overachiever—a perfectionist no matter the circumstances.

I now understood why telling people felt so important to me, as excruciating as it was. I had kept this secret for so long, even denying it to myself, and the secrecy had made me sick. Talking about it was the remedy, the cure. It neutralized the shame. The only way to heal now was to speak out loud what had been done to me—to say it over and over again, as loud as I could, looking directly into someone else's eyes. For so many years, these secrets, this truth, had lived inside me. Now I needed it outside of me. All those years, I'd had a tell. Now I needed *to* tell.

I knew, as with Lizzie, I would have to tell my parents in person. John and I arranged to visit them in Arizona, where they spent a lot of time at a house on a golf course in Phoenix that had belonged to my grandmother Novie. It was the place where I'd swum in a freezing-cold pool that my father didn't heat on principle, where Courtney and I had blasted Madonna from our jam box, where I'd been amazed to see grapefruit hanging from a tree, since you could see for miles in the Texas Panhandle, no tropical fruit in sight. The house in Arizona held a lot of history, and it was there that I would rewrite mine.

At the end of my weekly session with Lauren, she presented me with a deck of cards, each with a different animal. "What do you think—do you want to pull a card?" she said. "You've been working so hard. This will be fun."

The cards fanned out before me, face down, I tugged at several, finally pulling one at the back of the stack. I turned it over, face up.

"The earthworm?" I said incredulously. "After all the therapy and processing, journaling and reflecting—now I'm being compared to an earthworm? This feels like a cruel joke."

"Just a minute, Amy," Lauren said. "Let's not be so critical. Look at that card. What does it say?"

I read the card. "The earthworm feels small and insignificant, but it's an important part of the web of life. It can be hard to see the big picture, especially when you are down in the dirt, but please know that you matter. Your life has great purpose and meaning." I looked back at Lauren. "Sorry, I'm still stuck on the fact that I'm a worm. Not the inspiration I was hoping for." She smiled. "But I get it. This is where I am. I'm in the dirt, investigating every possible hole." And I knew I was going to have to stay there for a while.

ON THE FLIGHT TO Arizona, I was still practicing my delivery—thinking through what my parents could handle hearing—when I got a message from William. "I know today is a big day," he wrote. "Remember to put your feet on the ground and just breathe. There's nothing you can't do today." He sent along a quote from an Adrienne Rich poem that he loved: "There must be those among whom we can sit down and weep, and still be counted as warriors." That was exactly what I wanted: to know that I could cry and howl and grieve and not be seen as weak but be seen instead as someone who was fighting for survival. I tore a scrap of paper out of my notebook and wrote the passage down, slipping it into my pocket.

As we pulled up to my parents' house, I felt like my organs were frozen inside my body. "Heads-up, Mom called me last night," Lizzie texted me. "She asked if I knew why you guys were coming. She thought maybe John was thinking of making a career change or that you were going to upend the kids and move overseas. Just wanted you to know she's asking questions." I touched the scrap of paper in my pocket. *Just breathe.*

Making our way up the drive, I could see my mother was already standing on the edge of the curb under a palm tree to greet us, waving brightly.

"I made a cheese plate!" she said. "We're so happy you're here. Do you want to go over to the hotel and have lunch—or should we go for a walk?"

"Can we all sit on the patio and catch up?" I said. Suddenly I was as centered as I'd ever been. It was go time. I had to let this out. I had come here because the investigation couldn't continue until my parents knew the truth, but now that I was here, I could feel that it was about more than that: It was time they understood what I had been running from all these years. I'd kept it a secret for so long, and now I was finally freeing myself of that burden.

"That's a great idea," she said, but I could hear the hesitation in her voice; she knew something was up. She grabbed blankets so we could get cozy on the covered porch. I sat on the couch with John, my father sitting in a chair next to my mother, directly across from me. It felt forced and overly formal, but I needed to be able to look them in the eye as I addressed them.

"I have to tell you a story," I said slowly. "It's long, and very difficult to share with you." Both of them looked at me with concern and confusion. "It involves abuse that started in my childhood," I said. With that, they froze.

"Are you telling me that he hurt you?" my mother said as I began to speak about Mr. Mason. It was incomprehensible to her, as if she couldn't take it in. "But weren't you and Courtney friends with him? I thought you liked him." As I continued talking, she stood, gasping. "I need to get some water," she said. When she didn't come back, I followed her inside and found her curled up on the stone floor in the fetal position, sobbing. "Mom," I said, putting my hand gently on her back, "please get up and come back outside. I know this is all hard to hear, but I have to finish my story." I could barely get the words out. I felt outside of myself somehow, witnessing my mother, who loved me more than anything, having her heart broken. But to continue hiding what happened from her would be even worse. I had to believe this truth would set us both free, if only I could tell it.

Back on the patio, she wailed inconsolably. "Why did I let you walk home from school every day?" she cried. "I can't go on. I've failed as a mother." She sat next to me on the couch and gripped my hand. "Why didn't you tell me, Amy?" she asked. "We would have stopped it! We would have been there for you!"

"He told me that no one would believe me because I came from such a nice family," I said. "Telling you wasn't worth the risk."

She looked at me in shock. "And other people know about this already? Why didn't you come to us the second you remembered?"

"Because the secret was supposed to be kept from you," I said. "It's only now that I'm able to admit it, in this moment. It's taken this long."

John remained mostly silent for the hours we were talking, as the sun went down and the night grew cooler. He didn't need to speak; I could feel him supporting me, sitting next to me.

"I know that I need to pursue criminal charges against Mr. Mason," I said. "It's not that I need to see him in jail to feel validated, but I do need to know that other people are safe. That he can't hurt anyone else. To end the cycle of abuse."

"I'll go see the teacher tomorrow, if you want me to," my father said darkly. "You just tell me what you want me to do, Amy."

"What I need is for you to let me lead this process," I said. "And I know that's going to be hard for you, as the head of this family and as someone who likes to be in control. But I need to do this on my own time. It's something only I can do." I met my father's gaze. "Part of why I'm here now is because I need your help in Amarillo, on the ground there, to hold him accountable."

My father looked back at me, unblinking. I had been preparing for his reaction for so long. Would he say he didn't believe me? Would he worry about hurting the family reputation? Yet for all his rigidity and conservatism, for all the years he ruled with an iron fist, now he looked at me with tenderness.

"Amy," he said, "we will stand by you every step of the

way. We might have missed this in the first half of your life, but we won't miss a thing in the second."

IT WAS BRUTAL TO have these conversations, brutal to re-count it to the people who loved me most but hadn't seen it, but I could feel, as if compelled by forces beyond me, that I had to do it. No matter how ugly the truth was, it was better to be able to examine it under the light than to keep it tucked away in the basement. I had spent so many years hiding that to bare it all was liberating, even as it hurt all of us.

It was three in the morning when John and I finally went upstairs to crawl into bed. As we brushed our teeth, he looked over at me. "You left nothing out," he said.

"I couldn't," I said, resting my hands on both sides of the sink. "No more secrets."

IN THE MORNING, OVER breakfast, my mom still looked dazed. "Your father and I didn't sleep," she said. "Amy, I don't know anyone who anything remotely like this has ever happened to. This kind of thing just doesn't happen."

"Mom, it happened to *you*, too," I said gently. "With the milkman—remember?"

She looked at me, stunned. "I guess that's true. But I have to tell you, Amy"—she pushed the food around on her plate, then looked up at me—"I don't remember a lot of what you said to us last night. It's like I just couldn't take it in."

I held her gaze across the table. "It's okay, Mom," I said. "That's called dissociation." I sighed. "It's just how memory works."

8. KALI

The bald man on my laptop screen was seated at a desk. But as I squinted, I found myself focusing on the oil painting behind him. It was a familiar backdrop—it looked like Palo Duro Canyon, where I'd gone running as a girl. As he tilted his head to the side, I saw that it wasn't just a desert landscape but that there was something pulling the focus to the center of the painting: a prickly ball of thistle rolling through it—a tumbleweed.

I studied it. It was easier to focus on the painting than on this man, who was the newest addition to my legal team. The success of my case now rested in his hands. Cate had suggested that we find someone local to help us navigate the criminal justice system in Amarillo. But this man was a caricature. I could imagine him reclining in his brown leather desk chair, heels crossed at his ankles, wearing a giant pair of shitkicker boots. Everything about him, including his accent, called up the most triggering things from back home.

"Amy," Cate was saying, "I'm so glad to introduce you to Duke, the lawyer based in Amarillo who came recommended by your father. We've been talking about best course of action for your case and wanted you to meet directly."

"It's good to meet you, Amy," Duke said in a slow drawl. "Your dad called me about talking to you to see what could be done here. I've known your family a long time. I hope I can be helpful."

"Thanks, Duke," I said. "We wanted to bring you on board to help us navigate the local landscape." I looked at the tumbleweed again.

"Duke, as far as I can tell, the statute of limitations has changed over time such that Amy can pursue her case, but it would be great for you to verify that," Cate said. "And I'm hoping you can set the scene for us in Texas, because it's not my area of expertise, and there are always nuances with local law."

"I'll start working on that," Duke said.

"I've been looking into his past," I said. "We've just scratched the surface and no one else has come forward, but I'm moving forward regardless. I know what he did to me, and that's all that matters. Now we just need to assemble the pieces to start building a case."

"Well, one thing I wanna say is that you're gonna have to slow down," Duke said. "'Cause there's lots of things that have to happen here to line up."

"Oh, I grew up in West Texas," I said. "I know things move slowly down there. But I hope you'll get on board with me." Whether this was fair or not, Duke reminded me of so many of the men I'd grown up around. They were in charge, and I was not.

Not long after that first meeting, I was on the phone with my mom. "Your father just ran into Duke at lunch," she said excitedly.

She was telling me this so it would inspire confidence—but instead I felt like they were colluding, talking about me behind my back. Fury built within me. *Back to the western saloon days. I might as well side-saddle my horse and fasten my bonnet.*

"Well, that's completely inappropriate. I am an adult woman. Why is the lawyer I've hired, who I'm paying for, talking to my father without my involvement?"

"Oh, Amy, I don't think it was like that. I think they were just trying to be helpful—"

"I need to call Cate," I said. "This is insane."

I hung up the phone, incensed. I'd never had a temper before—I always put on a big smile, aiming to please—but lately I had been quick to anger. My fuse had shortened. I didn't know whom to trust and felt uneasy about handing everything over to another man in the place where it all happened. Yet I knew that I could not truly rest until Mason had been brought to justice—until there was some form of resolution.

"THAT'S KALI COMING OUT," Lauren said in our next session. "I can feel it."

"Who is Kali?" I asked.

"The Hindu goddess of divine feminine energy," Lauren said. "She possesses the power of both creation and destruction. They're two sides of the same coin."

"I'm feeling more destructive than creative right now," I said.

"Of course you are," she said. "But you have to be careful that you don't take everything down around you as you process this anger. Kali is so powerful, but used in the wrong way, that energy can do more harm than good."

More and more, all I wanted to do was burn things to the ground. I was angry: angry that I had to navigate this patriarchal culture to have any hope of getting justice; angry that, as a woman who could easily be dismissed as hysterical, I was responsible for carrying the burden of proof; angry that on some level I still felt like I'd betrayed my family by leaving this small town and never coming back, making me forever an outsider. The divide between me and the girl I'd been was so vast that all I could feel across it was rage. And so everything infuriated me, from the weeks it would take for Duke to respond to an email to his repeated characterization of me as a "victim."

"Duke, I am a *survivor*," I'd tell him, so much tension in my body I felt like I was about to pop a blood vessel. He never noticed that I corrected him.

BUT IN MY OWN house, it was becoming clearer that I was struggling. One evening, John turned to me. "Something interesting happened today with Gigi," he said. "She asked me if something happened to you."

I froze. "What did you say?" I asked.

"I said she should ask you," John said.

I should have known something like this was coming. Earlier in the week, she had come home complaining about a creepy store clerk; she and her friends were worried that he might abuse them, she said.

"Abuse you?" I asked.

"Yeah," Gigi said. "He was just really weird." She was only eleven.

"Did you feel safe?" I asked.

"No," she said. "Not at all. We left the store."

"That's so scary," I said. "But I'm glad you were with your friends, so there was someone there to see that he was being weird." I paused, collecting my words. "There's something important that I have to tell you, though. Yes, there will be strangers who make you feel uncomfortable. But sometimes, it's the people you're closest to who might try to take advantage of you."

"Mom," she said, annoyed. "What are you talking about?"

"Coaches," I said. "Teachers. Tutors. Clergy. Anyone who has repeated contact with you. Those are the people you should be more worried about. Not random people in stores." I took a deep breath. "But I'm sorry you had such a bad experience. And I'm glad you're paying attention."

"But Mom," she said, "those are the people I trust."

"That's what I'm saying," I said. "Sometimes people abuse your trust. And it's important for you to know that if anything bad happens, it's not your fault. And you can talk to me about it. Does that make sense?"

"Okay," Gigi said. But she only seemed more confused.

Now, as John revealed that she had asked him about me, I felt that I had revealed too much. "I think you're going to have to tell her," he said. "How do you feel about it?"

"I know you're right," I said. "But if I tell Gigi, I need to make a plan to tell all the kids. Julian's too young, but the older three." In the months that I'd been struggling, I was grateful that my older kids were teens who, for better or for worse, wouldn't notice if the sky fell so long as they still had their phones. John had continued to pick up the slack while I was attempting to reparent myself. He had done so without my having to ask, filling me in on lost retainers and sleepover plans so I never felt out of the loop.

Had my children felt this absence? I had no idea how anyone saw me anymore. John had gently told me that friends had expressed concern at how gaunt I'd become, but I felt disconnected from my own physical appearance. There was a part of me that hoped I would just disappear.

"Have you thought about how you want to have those conversations?" John asked.

"I've been working on it," I said. "It feels so raw, especially because the girls are around the age I was when I was abused. But kids can sense this stuff. I have to be honest with them. I just don't want to scar them in any way." I sighed. "As a parent, it would feel so good to be able to show them that there was some resolution. That I'd come out the other side stronger, and gotten justice."

"I don't know if they can wait for you to get justice," John said. "They're starting to sense that something's up."

"I just need a little more time," I said. "I can't tell them when it's all still such a mess. Isn't it a parent's job to have the answers? And I don't have any yet."

"It's your story to tell," John said. "You'll know when it's the right time."

A FEW DAYS AFTER my meeting with Duke, I sent along a recording of the statement I'd made for Cate and her team, describing in detail every incident of abuse that I could remember. Then I waited for him to review the recordings.

Days turned into weeks; I left word for him a handful of times but didn't hear back. Finally we were able to confirm another meeting. By the time the day arrived, I was irritated; the waiting had been agonizing.

"I'm sorry about all this," he said. "I did listen to the tape. I have a daughter, so it's very hard to hear." This made me soften toward him, but I was still annoyed that he'd been so impossible to reach. I worried he had taken the case only as a favor to my father, which made me feel sidelined, as though I didn't even matter. Couldn't he see that I was in distress? Or was I asking too much?

"So what are our next steps?" I asked.

"Well, it's important that we be patient, Amy, and not rush anything. I've been pokin' around at the DA's office, who now know about your case but not the details. They want you to talk to a detective. Are you willing to come down here and do it in person?"

"There's no chance I can come home right now," I said. The last thing I wanted to do was return to the scene of the crime. I hadn't been back to Amarillo since I'd recovered the memories; I wasn't sure if I'd ever go back. In my mind, I'd drawn an invisible boundary around the Texas Panhandle, and I would avoid it for as long as possible.

"Then a detective is going to call you to take your statement," Duke said. "A couple things I want to talk to you about before you do that. First of all, that lady who gave you the pill. I wouldn't mention her."

"Wait, what?" I said. "It was a psychedelic-assisted therapy session. This was in a controlled setting under expert supervision—"

"Sure," Duke said, "but people down here won't know about all that."

"Got it," I said, barely containing my frustration. "And what else?"

"You should make a time line of everything that happened," he said. "It will be helpful to have all the specifics in writing."

"I'll take the next week or so to work on that," I said.

"And one last thing," he said. "I know you mentioned there was one last incident of abuse, when you were in high school." In my mind's eye, I saw the tennis center and Mr. Mason waving to me on the curb as I pulled up in my blue Blazer. *One more time, for old times' sake?* "I'd leave that out," Duke said.

"Why?" I said. "It happened. Shouldn't I be completely honest?"

"There's so much here," he said. "You don't need it. It's going to be harder for a jury to understand why, at that age, you didn't just run away or tell someone."

"I just dissolved every time he came around me," I said. "That may be hard for you to understand. It didn't matter what age I was. He had complete power over me."

"I believe you," Duke replied. "It will just be harder to prove."

But did he believe me? Was I having to prove myself to my own lawyer? The thought was infuriating. Nothing made me spin out more than someone saying that they believed me— why *wouldn't* they? It felt as if there were an unspoken "but" at the end of the sentence. *I believe you, but why didn't you tell anyone? I believe you, but why did it take you so long to remember? I believe you, but weren't you on drugs?* I knew that these memories were real. My body knew what had happened to me. The way I'd shake when I'd tell my story; the way my eyes welled up with tears at the mention of Texas. And yet still I had no proof.

"Understood," I said. "I'll be expecting the detective's call."

A few days later, driving to pick up Gigi from a friend's house, my phone rang. I recognized the Amarillo area code. *Here goes.* I picked up.

"Hello, this is Sergeant Hank Jones. I'm calling for Amy Griffin?"

"Yes, hi—this is Amy," I stammered.

"I'm calling to see if I can find some time with you in the next week to ask you a few questions," he said. I pulled over.

"Let me just look at my calendar," I said. Then I wondered: Could he hear that I was in the car? "Sorry, I'm not looking at my phone while I'm driving," I said defensively. "I pulled over." *Why did you tell him that? He didn't accuse you of anything.* All it took was a male authority figure with a West Texas drawl, and I was falling over myself to prove that I'd done nothing wrong.

"Oh, don't worry, ma'am," he said. "I'm not worried about that in the least."

I listed some times for the call. "Is this over the phone or on video?"

"Phone is just fine, ma'am," he said. "I'll speak to you then. Have a nice weekend."

I rested my head on the steering wheel for a moment before pulling back onto the road. *This is it,* I thought. I had brought law enforcement into the conversation now. Things were falling into place, just as I had hoped. It was going to feel so good to be able to tell my kids that I'd brought my perpetrator to justice—that the world always rights itself, and the good guys win.

On a sunny afternoon a few days later, I sat in my bedroom and, over the course of two hours, relayed the story, in as much detail as possible, of what Mr. Mason had done to me. The detective listened intently, responding kindly with occasional words of affirmation.

"It still bothers me that my memories are incomplete," I said. "I wish I could remember more."

"It's actually the opposite," he said. "If you were able to give me a cohesive story of every detail that happened from start to finish, about something that happened over thirty years ago, I would find that unusual."

"Really?"

"I've been doing this a long time," he said. "That's just not how most survivors give their statements."

I took a deep breath. "Thank you," I said. He didn't have to say that he believed me—I knew that he did.

"This is one of the most credible calls I've had in all my years of doing this," he said. "I should have him in my office within the next few days."

"Really?" I said. "In your office?"

"Yup. Sometimes these guys just come right out and admit it. They can't live with themselves."

For the first time in months, I felt something unfamiliar— a bubble of hope within me that felt like it was filling me from the inside out. The police believed me; Mr. Mason might soon be in custody; then I could tell my children, and life would go back to normal. How validating it would be to know that Mr. Mason would not be able to hurt anyone else—that I was right and he was wrong. The world would take care of me. Things would work out.

All those months ago, William had told me that I had to take care of myself alongside my fight for justice. I had managed to do both at the same time. Now, by bringing Mr. Mason to justice, I'd be doing what was expected of me to protect others.

Hope—for the first time in a long time, I felt hope.

THE NEXT MORNING, MY phone rang while I was in the bathroom. Amarillo Police Department again. "Amy, this is Sergeant Jones calling," he said. I could hear in the tone of his voice that something was wrong. "I need to tell you something before we go any further."

What could have happened between yesterday and today? Reflexively I felt responsible. Surely I had done something wrong.

"I've been discussing this with my superiors all morning, and as far as I can tell, the statute of limitations has run out for your case," he said. He began listing numbers, years, and changes to the law. "The statute of limitations would have expired when you were twenty-eight," he said. "A few years after that, the law was changed such that there is no longer a statute of limitations in Texas. But because the law was changed after it had already expired on your case, incidents that predate the change to the law cannot be prosecuted criminally."

I froze, sliding down the bathroom wall to sit on the floor. "Amy?" he was saying. "Amy?" His voice sounded a million miles away. I held my hands to my face.

"I have to tell you something," I said. I could hear my voice trembling. "It happened in high school."

"I thought it happened when you were in middle school."

"There was one more incident that I didn't report," I said. I told him about the final time, at the tennis center.

"Why didn't you tell me this yesterday?"

I felt defensive, as if I'd done something wrong. "My lawyer told me not to mention that part of the story," I said. "He thought it wouldn't play well."

"Let me guess," the detective said. "He's a criminal defense attorney. He's thinking of you as the criminal, not as a survivor." I held my breath. "Amy, it would have been perfectly normal for you to freeze and do as this man told you to at sixteen."

I felt myself begin to cry. "Thank you for saying that," I said.

"So you were sixteen when it happened? It would have been four years after the abuse began?"

"Yes," I said. "That's right."

I heard him clicking his tongue. "I'm afraid that still leaves us a few years short of when the statute of limitations was changed. I'm just so sorry, Amy. We can't pursue a criminal case. There's nothing I would rather do than go after this guy, but we can't. The only way this case proceeds is if others come forward whose cases fall within the current statute of limitations."

Time seemed to slow down. It was everything I could do to mumble a "thank you" and hang up the phone.

What just happened?

The awareness grew slowly. *So . . . it's over? The law says there's nothing I can do?* I knew from talking to Cate that if I tried to bring charges in civil court, Mason could countersue me. I might end up spending the rest of my life in a West Texas courthouse just to prove a point.

There would be no justice.

How had we gotten this far before realizing the limits of the law? Wasn't that Duke's job—to know the laws in Texas? I felt rage burn inside my stomach, all directed at Duke.

I picked up the phone, feeling cold fury. Duke's receptionist answered. "I'm sorry, Mrs. Griffin, but he's away on a fishing trip," she said.

"It is so important that you find him," I begged. "Please, tell him to call me immediately."

When Duke called me back, a few hours later, my anger had only intensified. "The sergeant seems to think the dates don't work," I said.

"*We-ell*, remember, he's a detective and I'm a lawyer," he said. "I'll have to check on that."

"He seemed pretty confident," I said.

"Amy," Duke said in that long Texas drawl, "I'm taking the first vacation I've had in fourteen months. I'll be back in the office in ten days."

"Can you call the sergeant and talk to him?" I pleaded. "I feel like my life is hanging in the balance."

"*We-ell*, you'll have to wait until I'm home," he said. "I need you to be patient."

I gripped the phone. If he told me to be patient one more time, I was going to hurl it across the room. Kali's claws were out. None of her creation. Only her destruction.

I hung up and called Cate. "Cate," I said, "Duke told me I have to wait until he's back for answers. I can't wait ten days to know what's happening here."

"I'm just as frustrated as you are," she said. "I can't give you those answers. That's why we hired Duke. But he simply isn't responsive."

"I'm not angry at you," I said.

"You should be," she said. "I feel like I'm letting you down here."

"Isn't there anything more we can do?" I pleaded. I had

convinced myself that the only way I'd ever be able to move forward after having unearthed the trauma of having been abused would be to get some kind of justice, whatever that meant. I could feel the possibility of that slipping away.

"We'll find another Texas-based lawyer who can check whether the detective's math is correct," she said. "We should have a final answer soon."

IN SESSION WITH LAUREN, I spat venom.

"Is it possible that Duke really is on your team?" she proposed. "That he's trying to be helpful?"

"No!" I yelled. "On my team? Are you kidding me?" Whose side was she on? Even her asking the question made me feel alone and misunderstood. "I'm telling you—I have *never* felt supported by this person! He epitomizes everything I ran from in Texas! Don't tell me to be patient! He's supposed to be *helping* me! By the way, he *still* hasn't gotten back to me! I hope he's caught a lot of fish by now!"

"Amy, I understand that you don't feel supported. But let's think about what being supported looks like to you."

"Frankly, I don't feel supported by anyone right now!" I yelled. I knew that I was being childish, but I didn't care. There was a twelve-year-old within me who still felt neglected, and she was howling to be seen.

FINALLY CATE CALLED ME back. "We found a lawyer in Houston who did some research, and unfortunately the detective was right," she said. "A child molester serving a sentence in a Texas jail recently had his conviction overturned by appealing on the grounds that his crime was committed before the statute of limitations had been extended, such that the old statute of limitations applied."

"What?" I said. "I can't even follow that."

"I can send you the cases," she said. "Basically, the crimes were reported too late. The statute of limitations had already run out by the time they changed the law. It's a loophole."

I slumped to the floor. It was the same spot where I'd curled up months ago, where I'd thrown the soap across the room the night after my first MDMA session, knowing that my life had just changed forever.

But had it? I had remembered everything; I had shattered the glass case I had constructed inside me, but it had changed nothing. I'd gone in a circle, right back to where I'd started. I felt more powerless than ever.

HAD I LEFT ANY stone unturned? I racked my brain, reviewing the notes from my conversations with Cate about the investigation. What about Allie—the girl who had seen something creepy on a school trip, the girl the investigators couldn't track down?

I enlisted my mother to get me her phone number, which was no small feat; she had to ask a friend of a friend to ask her daughter, all of which would raise questions as to why the number was needed in the first place, but I was done worrying about rocking the boat. "Just tell them it's for me," I said. "I don't care if it gets people talking."

On the phone, Allie's voice was a breath of fresh air. "Of course I remember Mr. Mason," she said. "God, he was such a creep."

"You do?" I said, my voice rising incredulously. *Hope!* "What do you remember?"

"Well, that he was specifically creepy about *you,* for one thing," she said. "I have such a clear memory of him standing really close to you, talking, in the hallway."

"Yes!" I said. My heart surged. Finally, somebody with a memory as vivid as mine! "I didn't realize anyone else noticed! He searched me out to talk all the time!"

"He was always staring at you," she said. "At the time, I didn't think much of it, but also, I definitely noticed it. It felt like you were the only thing he saw."

"I can't believe you remember that," I said.

"Oh, it stuck with me because there was something so weird about him," she said. "Even on the first day of class, he was joking around with me with this huge creepy smile— like, so passive-aggressive. I even remember telling my mom about it. My forty-six-year-old brain can see that he was flirting with me and testing me."

"Is there anything else?" I asked. "What happened on the trip he chaperoned?"

"That was so unsettling," she said. "For some reason he had to drive us out there, me and Emily, and the way he pulled up fast and jumped out—kind of hyper and silly—it was like he was picking up two girls for a date or something. In the car I remember him staring at Emily's crotch, looking back at me in the rearview mirror, then looking back down at her. I had this terrible feeling, like we were being kidnapped. The whole thing just felt really unsafe."

"What happened that night?" I said. I was trembling. "Didn't something happen later on that night, that you told somebody about?"

"Oh, yes," she said. *This is it,* I thought. *This is how I'm going to get him.* "That night all of the girls were in sleeping bags in the main living room. I woke up in the middle of the night, and he was standing in the room. He wasn't moving." Chills ran down my body. "There was some light on, because I could see him clearly. It was silent in the room—everybody else was asleep. I didn't even lift my head because I didn't want him to know I was awake. My heart was pounding out of my chest. He was staring at me with no expression on his face. Looking straight into my eyes. I closed my eyes and turned my head to the right, and the next thing I remember, it was morning." She exhaled heavily. "I never told anyone. I should have jumped up and screamed at the top of my lungs. I wish I could do that now."

"So he was just looking at you?" I said. My heart sank. I felt sorry for what Allie had experienced and that, like me, she had kept it a secret. But I was so desperate for someone to confirm my experience, I'd hoped she would remember something that could bolster my case. Nothing she described was criminal.

"It's so strange," she said. "I literally just started thinking about all of this a few months ago. I mean, there must be someone else who saw something. Someone else it happened to."

"I don't think there is," I said, wanting to cry. "I've talked to everyone."

"Well, you know how small towns work," Allie said. "People want to sweep things under the rug, pretend like everything's fine. Nobody wants to talk about what might be really going on. Everything has to look perfect."

I knew she was right. When was I going to accept it? If

anyone else had been subjected to the same abuse, they were never coming forward. I was alone, fighting a battle I had already lost.

TALKING TO LAUREN, I spun out. "I had believed that I'd be able to hold him responsible, and now I am mourning that dead end. And I have this family trip next week—"

"Oh, for your dad's birthday?" She looked concerned. "That's a lot to be asking of yourself right now. Are you sure you're up for it?"

"We've been planning this for a year," I said. It was my father's seventieth birthday, and I had organized a trip to the Smoky Mountains in Tennessee with my whole family to celebrate. It was the first time the family would be all together since I'd told them individually about what I'd been processing. "I want to go."

But when John and I landed in Knoxville, I was still fuming about Duke, who had come to represent everything I thought was wrong with the Texas culture I'd grown up in: men doing favors for one another; women helpless on the sidelines; legal loopholes that make it impossible for the law to actually protect anyone; bureaucratic red tape. Yet I was desperate for my family to enjoy this trip, and I didn't want what I was going through to ruin my father's birthday, so I decided to lock all my anger and grief away—to put it out of my mind for the long weekend.

For the duration of the trip, I managed to avoid the subjects of politics and religion. Instead, everyone stuck to the script: college football, the delicious food, and the beautiful scenery. At his birthday dinner, toasting us, my dad was genuinely moved. "It means so much to me to have all of us here together," he said, getting choked up. It was so rare to see him emotional; it brought me back to the tears I'd seen in his eyes in that middle-school auditorium.

But something was shifting within me by the end of the weekend. I was weary of holding it all together and pretending everything was fine. On a hike the final morning, I cruised for a fight, tiptoeing into conversations about politicians I loathed and reproductive rights in my family's home state to see if I could get a rise out of anyone. The personal felt newly political, and vice versa. Kali was swinging from the branches, walking alongside me.

"So how are you really?" Lizzie said, sidling up next to me as we returned to the base of the mountain. "I didn't want to ask in front of everyone else, but I've been so worried about you." The question, well-intentioned as it was, infuriated me.

"How am I?" I snapped. "I'm not good. I need someone to take this away from me."

"I know what you're going through must be so hard," she said. "I'm devastated too."

"*You're* devastated?" I howled. "You have no idea what I've been through! It didn't happen to you! It happened to *me!*" I did not recognize the sound of my own voice, a primal wail. "Can you step outside the bubble of Texas for one second to see what I see? Don't you ever walk down the street and realize that you don't have control over your own lives there? Lizzie, your daughters will have fewer freedoms there than we did growing up! How can you not demand bodily autonomy for your girls! Do you know how valuable the work is that you do around the house? Jesus, you do everything for your kids, your husband, your family—and you don't even have free will over your own body!"

"You think we're all stupid because we live in Texas," Lizzie said.

"No, I just want you to look around and recognize how the culture we grew up in allowed this all to happen!" I screamed.

My mom looked shocked. She kept shaking her head from side to side. She had never seen me in a state like this. "You are so angry," she said. "So angry. I pray you get rid of this anger and find happiness."

"I pray for that too, Mom, but the anger is part of it!" I yelled. "Don't you see I'm the twelve-year-old now who needs the support I didn't get back then? Can you just support me, knowing that I'm as fragile as I was then, when I was a twelve-year-old who was being raped and beaten? Would you like me to put on a fucking smile?"

She winced. She hated it when I cursed. "What you've been through is horrible," she started to say, then she put her hands to her face.

"How can you go about your lives knowing that women are being stripped of their rights?" I shrieked. I whirled around to face my mother. "What if I had gotten pregnant in middle school, Mom? What then?"

"Amy, this is the worst thing that has happened in any of our lives," she said. "This is unthinkable as a mother. I wish it had been me and not you. And we will do anything if you just tell us what you need."

"I don't know what I need," I screamed, tearing at my hair.

Exhausted, defeated, hearing the words out loud, I realized it was true. I had clung to this hope of justice because I had believed that it would right the wrong, somehow. That it would deliver me a perfect ending to this terrible story.

But there was no such thing as perfect.

. . .

I KICKED AND SCREAMED in the car on the way to the airport, like a toddler having a tantrum. My mother and sister stared at each other, not knowing what to do. I had completely lost control. I could not pretend anymore that anything about this was tolerable. I was a burning inferno, a ball of pure anguish.

Finally, the storm within me passed. I sat numbly, watching the green hills of Tennessee disappear through the window. I was drained of all feeling.

I felt like the earthworm on the card I'd pulled—on the ground, in the darkness. I had never felt so small.

I did not know how I was going to crawl out of this hole.

9. PERFECT

Back in New York, the sinus infection that I'd been try-ing to keep at bay got the best of me. I sulked around my apartment on antibiotics. Yet in my exhaustion was an eerie sense of calm. I had laid myself bare in front of my family, finally expressing what I had kept inside for so long—hoping that some element of my ragged desperation would resonate with them. It was cathartic, and I didn't regret it. I told my mother and sister that I needed some time to pro-cess, and they gave it to me.

But none of it changed the fact that I had no further re-course against Mr. Mason—that the justice I'd long imag-ined would bring me peace would not come to pass. I did not want to have to explain to my children that because of a bu-reaucratic loophole, the man who had hurt me all those years ago was still out there, free to abuse others—and that I could do nothing to stop it. As a mother, this was the deepest pain: How could I tell my children I could protect them if they knew I couldn't protect myself?

"I don't know how much longer you can wait to tell them," John said to me.

"I know," I said. "But there's someone I think I need to talk to first."

I ASKED CLARA, THE teacher at my daughters' school, to meet with me—not at school but at my office, where we could talk privately. "I need to ask your advice about something to do with my girls," I said after we sat down. "But first, I guess it makes sense to tell you what I've been going through. Are you open to me sharing something personal?" I pressed my hand to my throat, where I could feel my heart beating. "I feel I should warn you that it's a lot."

Clara assured me that she wanted to hear what I had to say. But after I'd spoken only a few sentences, I realized the look on her face was not just one of sadness but also one of familiarity. I realized why I'd always felt connected to her, even without articulating it. "Oh, Clara," I said. "You too?" Something about this truth rattled me to my core. I fell to my knees and reached for her hands, clasping them in mine. In an instant it hit me, the magnitude of this problem, the omnipresence of it—that it was all around me, and so much bigger than me or Clara. That there were so many of us carrying this same secret. "I'm so sorry. So deeply sorry. This must be so triggering for you. I had no idea."

"It went on for much of my childhood," Clara said. She

barely blinked, sitting up straight in her chair. "My husband is the only other person who knows."

"Have you done therapy to work through it?"

"I went once," she said. "But I just put it away in the back of my brain. Even though I'm sure it's part of why I do what I do—why I stand in front of a classroom full of girls every day, knowing that, statistically, something is happening to one in three of them."

One in three. It was too horrific to bear.

"It's so common," I said, "but we never talk about it. Which is why I need to talk to my girls and tell them my story. But how do I do it?"

Clara nodded. "You have to tell them the complete truth," she said. "I've watched your girls grow up. They're smart. Let them be your teachers." She had made a career of understanding how teens think, knowing what they could and couldn't handle at different developmental stages. If there was one person I could trust as to whether my girls were ready to hear what I had to tell them, it was she.

But as we sat there talking, I realized I was still resisting what I knew I had to do. The problem wasn't that my girls weren't ready. It was that I wasn't.

LATER THAT DAY, I caught up over the phone with Olivia. She didn't hold back. "What has this pursuit of justice really been about for you, Amy?" she said softly. "It's not about your daughters. It's about a little girl who was told: *No one will believe you.* So you've been on a quest to prove the man who said that to you was wrong. To make the world believe you. And like you do with everything else in your life, you've been trying to create a perfect outcome." I stopped walking and paused in front of a park bench, taking in what she was saying. I sat down and bowed my head to listen. "But this was never about arriving at a perfect outcome," Olivia said. "It was never about proof. It was only ever about you with you. You trusting you. What you need—what you've always needed—is just for *you* to know it. For you to show that little girl that you believe her. That she can trust you—that you can trust you to take care of you."

"But how do I do that?" I asked. "How do I show her that?"

"By being vulnerable with the people who love you most," Olivia said. "That was the thing you have always been afraid to do. So you tried to be perfect. Now you have the chance to show your girls what vulnerability looks like. You have the chance to show them who you really are."

It struck me, again, that my girls were the same age I'd been when I was abused. They were mirrors of me and for me. They had been the night when Gigi told me she felt like she didn't know me, and they were now. I saw so much of myself in them that to tell them what happened almost felt like I was breaking the news to my own childhood self. I was terrified that my trauma would traumatize them, that it would alter the course of their lives in some terrible way. Yet I knew that I needed to tell them. I needed them to listen in a way that I had never asked my children to listen before. The role reversal terrified me.

But what would it have been like, at that age, to have conversations that were that honest, with anyone, let alone with one of my parents? That, I thought, would have been true freedom—a kind of freedom that nobody could ever take away, a kind of authentic freedom that wasn't about control but about abandon. Letting go of the need to control. This was the gift I wanted to give my children.

I HAD LEARNED EARLY on that, with kids, difficult conversations were often best had in a casual, offhand way—in a car, or side by side at a diner—so I went to pick up Gigi from a sleepover with a plan to take her out for ice cream. I wanted to tell her first, since she had been the one to ask John if something had happened to me. Then I would tell the others in rapid succession. Walking there, I found myself spinning about how the conversation would go. She was eleven—would she understand? But I had to remember I was doing this for the connection—to break down the walls that she had so astutely identified all those months earlier when she'd told me I was there but not there.

"Mom, look at my nails!" Gigi squealed as she met me on the street. "We painted them pink last night."

"You really did," I said, glancing at her hot-pink nails. At least they weren't scarlet red, which would have been considered inappropriate for a girl her age when I was growing up. "Want to go for a smoothie?" There was a market a few blocks away. I looked down at the white lines of the crosswalk and reached for her hand. She was old enough now that she wouldn't usually let me hold it, but she must have been able to feel my energy because she clasped my fingers in hers.

"Gigi," I said as we walked, "do you remember asking Dad if something happened to me?"

"Yeah," she said, "a few weeks ago. He said I needed to

ask you because it was your story to tell, not his." She looked at me. "Did something happen?" she asked. "Do you have a story?" We entered a health food store that had a smoothie bar, weaving between aisles of artisanal chips and vegan ice cream.

"I do," I said. "Do you want to hear it?" We reached the line to order, which snaked around the back of the store, harried moms with toddlers in tow and a pack of twentysomethings carrying yoga mats.

"Mom, were you raped?" she asked. My heart stopped. I wanted to run. I looked around frantically: Who had heard? But before I could spiral, I knew I had to answer her.

"Yes," I said. "This line is really long—let's go to the ice-cream place instead."

"Mom, did it happen more than once?" Gigi asked.

"Yes," I said, "it happened more than once. Come on—let's go." I felt like I was hovering outside my own body as we made our way out of the store back onto the street.

"Mom, how old were you?" she asked.

"Twelve," I said. "Gigi, I was twelve."

Her face crumpled. "Wait," she said, "you were twelve? How is that possible?" She began to cry. "I can't believe that this happened to you."

Stay with it, I said to myself. *Don't dissociate. You can handle this.*

We entered an ice-cream parlor. She stood behind me, tears in her eyes, while I ordered—two scoops of moose tracks in a cone for her, none for me. My stomach was in knots. Afterward, we sat down on a bench outside and continued talking. Her ice cream went soft in the sun as we spoke.

"This is the hardest thing I've ever heard," she said. "Does this have anything to do with your job? Like how you're always working with other women who have companies?"

"You're five steps ahead of me," I said. "I never even really thought about that. But you're probably right. I guess because somebody made me feel really powerless a long time ago, it feels good to help other women find their power."

"Did you have any health problems after?" she asked. I paused. Her tone was so kind and loving; it felt as though she instinctively knew how to talk to survivors.

"I'm just now realizing how my body absorbed what happened to me," I said. I took a deep breath. "Gigi, there's something important I have to tell you. Do you remember that difficult conversation we had a few months ago, when we were sitting on your bed?"

She nodded.

"You and Gracie told me that you didn't really know who I was. You said, 'Mom, you are nice, but you are not real.' You remember that?"

She nodded again. I felt tears spilling out of my eyes. "I had been keeping this a secret for so long. But you helped me see that I needed to face it. You helped me realize that I needed to be honest with myself." My voice cracked. My heart was so full it was nearly unbearable—with love and gratitude for my daughter and for how she had brought me to this place. "And in being honest with myself, I could be more open with you and Gracie and your brothers. So I want to thank you for that." Her ice cream had melted to mush. I looked her straight in the eye, willing her to understand how much stronger I'd become because of her.

"So what are you going to do now?" she asked.

"Well, I was working on pursuing legal action against the man who raped me," I said. "But it turns out that I can't. It's very disappointing for me, because I wanted to be able to tell you that he could never hurt anyone else ever again. I wanted to tell you that I had solved the problem, that I'd taken care of it. But that's not what happened."

"Oh, I didn't mean like that," Gigi said. "I mean, how are you going to get better?"

I was caught off guard. "There's so much I've been doing to heal," I said. "Trying to slow down. Taking a bath every day. Feeling the sunlight on my face. Trying to notice things, even little things, like the colors of the leaves changing and the sound of them crunching under my feet. Have you noticed I've been going for a lot of walks lately?"

"I think so," she said. "And you're not running anymore."

"That's right," I said. "I'm not."

THE NEXT NIGHT, I took Gracie to dinner, just the two of us. We went to a dimly lit restaurant in the neighborhood that she loved. The room was almost empty—all the better, I thought, for what I was about to share with her. Gigi had been asking questions and had teed up the conversation for me, but for Gracie, this would be coming entirely out of left field. Grace was thoughtful and ambitious; she was so much like I had been at thirteen.

I positioned us at the table with care—her back to the restaurant, me facing out, so if she became emotional, the whole room wouldn't notice. We caught up on what was happening on her volleyball team and how her friends were doing. When we fell into silence, I said I had something dif-

ficult to share with her. Then I told her. There was one candle on the table between us, which flickered as I spoke. I
could feel her absorbing what I said; there was no judgment
in her expression. She was so steady. It felt as if she were
wrapping a blanket around my shoulders.

"This must be the hardest thing in the world to talk
about," she said. "You must have tucked this away in the
back of your brain for so long."

I nodded, surprised and impressed by how perceptive
she was. "Do you have any questions?" I asked. "You can ask
me anything."

"No, no, I get it," she said. "It's like how with generational
trauma you can feel something is there without knowing
what it is."

I looked at her. The fact that she was already aware of that
language was astonishing. "How do you know that term?" I
said.

"Mom, you may not realize this, but I deal with a lot of
stuff with my friends," she said. "I learned how trauma can
occur again and again if you don't break the cycle by acknowledging it."

I shook my head. "That is amazing," I said, "and makes
me feel so hopeful for your generation."

"I'm going to say something that I think might hurt your
feelings, but I'm going to say it anyway," she said.

"Go ahead."

"It's just that I've never really felt like I have known anything about your life," she said. "Like, I know about Dad, and
what happened with his sister, but with you—I just always
thought you were perfect. Sometimes I tell people that you're
so perfect, I don't know how I can ever be like you."

There was that word again—"perfect." It was a word that held a lot of charge for me. For years, when someone described me or my life that way, I'd reject or deflect the characterization. "I don't know what perfect even means," I'd say. The word felt crass. I never wanted anyone to notice my quest for perfection or to call me out for it. I'd always try to be like a duck: seeming to glide across the water effortlessly but frantically paddling my feet beneath the surface in order to stay afloat. I'd worked so hard to keep everyone happy, to do right by everyone, to never let the ball drop. I was always the first to volunteer, the first to deny my own needs to ensure someone else's comfort. But where had that gotten me? All that running had left me ragged—"nice but not real," as Gigi had said. I didn't want to model that for my daughters. I'd never want them to feel they couldn't truly be themselves.

I thought, again, about Olivia's wise words—how I'd focused on the external in this quest for perfection. I had wanted perfect justice, perfect confirmation, a perfect resolution. Now I wanted to let that go.

"I'm not perfect," I said. "And I don't want you to feel like I expect you to be. I know you're already under so much pressure, being a teenager in New York City. I don't want you to feel it from me, too." I paused, finding my words. "I know it's a lot to ask of you. But I'm hoping that you can bear with me, as your mom, as I continue untangling all this. There are ways I have parented you that are about control, and perfectionism, that don't serve either of us. And I'm sorry if you've ever felt any of that. But I'm realizing, more and more, that it's the painful, messy, complicated things that we need to go through together. Those are the things that make up a life."

Gracie reached across the table and took my hand in hers. "Well, now I understand why you thought you had to be perfect," she said. Of course my children didn't want me to be perfect—they wanted me to be reachable. That was exactly what Gigi had been trying to tell me that night when we argued in her bedroom. My vulnerability was not a weakness. It was the greatest gift I could give them.

JACK, WHO WAS SIXTEEN, was next on the list. It was important that my kids hear it from me, not from one another, so I knew I needed to keep the momentum going. A day after telling Grace, I asked Jack if we could have dinner one on one.

"I have a bonfire with friends tonight," he said.

"Early dinner?" I said.

As I sat across from him at the table, feeling buoyed by my conversations with my girls, he slathered a roll with butter. "So," he said, chewing, "what are you gonna order?"

"I'm glad we got this time alone," I said. I looked around the crowded restaurant, wondering if anyone I knew was there and whether they could overhear me. "I'm really proud of you for everything you're doing—I hope I tell you that enough."

"Uh-huh," he said. "I think I'm gonna get a steak."

"I wanted us to have dinner so I could tell you something about my life," I said. "I've told your sisters this in the last two days, and I'll tell Julian when he's a little bit older." As I told Jack the story, in a matter-of-fact way, he looked distressed. "Wow," he said, "that's really intense. I'm sorry. Are you okay now?"

"Yes," I said. "I'm trying to be. I've been working through the past. In case you felt that I was less present in the last few months, this is what I've been processing, and I wanted you to know that."

He reached for another piece of bread and scooped out the last bit of butter.

"Do you want to ask me anything?" I said.

"Nope," he said. "I'm good. I'm just glad you're okay."

I felt the corners of my mouth turn up, something resembling a smile. We had connected. It was enough.

I HAD TOLD EVERYONE who mattered most to me, pierced the blister of every secret, torn down everything that needed to be dismantled. There was only one more thing that I knew I had left to do—something I had been putting off for months. Something inside me told me that I needed to keep going with the MDMA therapy. But could I bear what I would find in another session? Olivia had never pressured me about it, but when I told her I thought I was finally ready, I could sense that she was glad I was returning to the medicine.

The day of the session, she sat across from me on the couch. "I'm hoping this brings you more resolution," she said in her gentle, accented voice. "Remember to be compassionate with yourself. You don't have to go in looking for anything. What you need to know, you'll find."

I nodded.

"One reason we do this work is so we can face whatever it is that we need to face," she said. "So we can live *with* what we've been through, instead of living *from* it."

I took the pill. How funny that just a few months earlier, I had been stricken with anxiety and shame about taking a drug, especially one that was illegal. I had always associated the taking of drugs with loss of control. And in some way, that was exactly what it had given me. I no longer felt the same need to control everything in my life—that rigidity that I'd felt since I was a teenager had simply vanished.

"Remember, Amy," she said, "we are so much more than what has been done to us."

As the familiar warmth of the MDMA settled in my chest, the first thing I saw was my mother, holding my hand. My heart melted. My hair was in perfect Princess Leia buns— one of many hairstyles that my mom had learned over the years while I sat at the foot of her bed—and I was holding a drawing of a rainbow with stick-figure children underneath it. I was eight years old.

"I'm with my mom," I said. "I love this memory." It was such a relief to not immediately be transported into something horrific and to be shown something that predated middle school. I could feel my mom's pride in me, and her love, deep and unwavering. It was a perfect love, one that had nothing to do with my accomplishments—a love that was a birthright, not something that had to be earned.

How loved I was—how loved I had always been. I thought about John, about friends from home, about my parents and my children. How good it felt to love and be loved, not for anything I had done but for who I was.

Then I was back in the classroom. Mr. Mason and I were circling each other on opposite sides of a desk, like a dance. It was late in the day; I could tell from the way the afternoon sunlight cut through the shades and how the light hit the countertops. He sat me up on the counter, pulled a desk up behind him, and sat on it. Within an instant, both of his hands were inside me.

I looked at the door that led to the hallway. There was a single glass panel in it, as there were in all the doors, but as with most classrooms, this one had been covered with a piece of fabric. If the window hadn't been covered, this wouldn't be happening, but I was glad that it was covered because I was so ashamed. "If I go back to that school some-day and there's no window in the doorway like I remem-bered, then that gives me an out," I said to Olivia. "Maybe I'm just making it up."

"Trust yourself," she said softly.

Then I was back in the bathroom, remembering it again, the way I had in the first two sessions. "Olivia," I said out loud, "I can't spend any more time in this bathroom. But I'm also scared to leave it. Scared that if I leave it, I'll forget what hap-pened here again. I'm scared to let it go, but I also don't want anyone else to ever have to be here." I sighed. "I want to take control of this memory," I said. "I want to change the story."

"It's your decision," Olivia said. "You get to decide."

"What if I blow it up?" I said.

I imagined the bathroom exploding like a giant disco ball. The doors of the bathroom stalls breaking up into tiny shards, then the tiled walls, then the mirrors. Glass shooting through the air, prismatic. The walls where mirrors had once hung no longer a painful reflection, no longer the tile that I'd clung to on the cold floor. I imagined the door blow-ing wide open.

"Is it okay to do that?" I asked Olivia. "To blow the whole place up?"

"Whatever you want," she said.

I imagined the sinks exploding, the remaining walls, until the only thing left was one wall with a window that was open, letting the light in. It was that light that I'd clung to as I lay on the bathroom floor, the light that I'd looked toward when what was happening felt unbearable. I was so relieved that the window was still there—that I could still see the sunlight. Then I imagined that window exploding too, letting in even more light.

The only thing left was the door. But instead of blowing it up, I imagined myself opening it and walking right out. In my imagination, the bathroom was gone. Now something new could be rebuilt in its place. Like Kali—destruction and creation, two sides of the same coin.

"DESTROYING THAT BATHROOM WAS really important," Lauren said. "What was that like for you? What did it mean?" It was a few days after my session, and I'd finally gotten enough perspective to process what I'd seen and experienced.

"I think it was a kind of resolution," I said. "I know it wasn't real, obviously—I could feel as it was happening that it was a fantasy—but I think in some way it allowed me to feel like some part of this can be over for me." I hesitated, ready to ask a question that I never thought I would ask. "Lauren," I said, "when is it okay to just put it down?"

"To put what down?"

"This," I said. "All of this. Trauma. Abuse. The past." I made air quotes. "*The work.*"

"You can put it down whenever you want, Amy," Lauren said. "It may continue to come up for you, of course, but you have some choice in how much space it takes up in your life."

"I guess I can pick it up again at some point," I said. "But I want to look forward, not backward. It's not that I'm afraid to look back because I'll see what's chasing me—I'm done living that way. I just don't want this to be the biggest thing in my life. There's so much more that I care about. My family, friends, my career, myself—I know this is a part of me, but I also don't want it to feel like it's *all* of me."

"Then put it down," Lauren said. "Allow yourself to put it down and see what happens."

LATER THAT NIGHT, AFTER my therapy session, I knocked on Gracie's door to find her getting dressed to head out for the evening. Clothes were strewn about her bedroom, fast fashion that had arrived in the apartment covertly, in brown boxes. It all always looked the same to me: black or pink, gauzy and synthetic. I could never tell what was a top and what was a skirt—it was all so tiny.

Things had been different when I was growing up. My mom had taught me how to put my hands straight down by my sides in front of the mirror once I'd gotten dressed before heading to a party. If my fingertips were longer than the hem of my skirt, then it was too short and I'd wear something else.

Why did she insist on that? I wondered. For the same reason that we, as parents, do anything. We want to keep our children safe. This is an evolutionary response as biologically ingrained as our own survival. I had always done that the best way I knew how, as had my mother. It came from a place of love.

And yet all the love in the world hadn't been enough to

keep me safe. There were predators from whom she had not been able to protect me. The length of my hem hadn't made a difference. So why did I care now about what Gracie wanted to wear? All those forms of control that I'd learned growing up hadn't kept me out of danger. I thought back to when I got my car for the first time and how free I felt, sailing down the open highway. Now I understood that I had mistaken control for freedom. The real way to keep my children safe wasn't to control them. It was to have an honest relationship with them. That was how I could set myself—and them—free.

Gracie used to try to run past me to the elevator, hoping that I wouldn't see what she was wearing. But our relationship was different now that I'd told her my story. I stood in her open doorway, watching her look at herself in the mirror.

She was wearing a pair of shredded jeans and a tube top, skin exposed, and was lacing up a pair of chunky black combat boots.

"Text me when you're on your way home," I said.

She nodded. "What do you think?" she said, turning to me.

"You look awesome," I said.

III. REBECOMING

10. FOUNDATION

"The school is sinking."

I was standing in my kitchen, on the phone with my mother.

"What?" I asked. "What do you mean, the school is sinking? Is that a metaphor?"

"Something about the foundation at Navarro," she said. "They're going to have to demolish the entire school and rebuild it."

"I don't know what to say," I said. "When is that happening?"

"Soon," she said. "I didn't know if you might want to see it before they tear it down. I know it's been such a long time since you've been home."

The old me would have lashed out at the suggestion. I

would have insisted that I was never coming back to Texas or used it as an opportunity to remind her how many terrible things had happened there. But instead I paused, considering.

"I'm just not sure," I said. "Coming home would be a big step. But I really miss being with you all. And I am dying for a bean burrito from Taco Villa."

"We miss you so much," my mom said. "We'd love to have you visit. Hey, I need another book recommendation from you. I finished *The Body Keeps the Score*."

"You did?" I said, excited.

"Oh, yes," she said. "All your back problems and hip surgeries—so much of it makes sense now. Your body was hanging on to so much. Reading it helped me process, too."

I smiled and closed my eyes. "Mom, really?" I said. "That means so much to me."

It had been two years since our trip to Tennessee for my dad's birthday. As the time passed, I began to understand what I'd felt I needed back in those days when I was out on a limb and needed "support." I had wanted so badly for others to see what had happened to me; I thought that would validate me, in the same way I had always sought external validation. But the confirmation and justice I'd been seeking weren't things I could get from the outside world. They were things I had to find within myself. In time I realized that where I needed to put my energy was my relationships, and so I had, starting with my family back home in Texas.

Lizzie and I hardly spoke for the better part of a year, even though I knew she desperately wanted to be there for me. But I needed some distance in order to heal; it was a great act of love that she gave it to me. Eventually, I came to see that I had been looking for someone to blame, and Lizzie was an easy target. My parents had given her so much emotional energy; irrationally, I believed that if more attention had been paid to my needs, I would not have been abused. I'd needed a safe place to put that anger, and there was no one safer to me than my sister. But I could see now just how misdirected the anger was.

With my parents, too, there were complicated feelings that I needed to unpack. I was angry with them for missing it, and angry, too, that because they were so shattered by my revelations, I felt responsible for their feelings, instead of getting to have my own. This was the secret at its core: I had always believed that if my parents knew about the abuse, they'd be crushed—and that somehow I'd be to blame. Mr. Mason had convinced me that my parents wouldn't love me anymore if I told; all this time, I had believed him. Now I had to allow my parents to show up for me in the ways that they did best.

It was my father who stepped in when Duke remained missing in action for several months after the case imploded; I wondered if he'd blown away like the tumbleweed in his painting. "I've called repeatedly and sent multiple letters, but he won't respond to me," Cate said. "I think we're at an impasse."

"I just want the rest of the retainer returned so I don't feel like this is still hanging over my head," I said. I knew instinctively what to do.

"I'll handle it," my dad said when I explained the situation to him. I understood that in the natural order of Amarillo, this was the only way I could close the loop, and I also understood that this was a gift I was giving to my father: that he would have the opportunity to parent me, even if it had to be with my own lawyer. Within a week, my dad had been to Duke's office to pick up a check for the unused portion of the retainer. I tried not to dwell on the fact that Duke had ignored both me and my female attorney for months when he responded to my father immediately. I regretted the time I'd wasted painstakingly gathering facts and consulting with lawyers, but I knew it was in the past—there was no use continuing to ruminate on it.

In reconnecting with my family, I had softened toward my home state. Rachel reminded me how many good people were still back in Amarillo, even if I wasn't entirely ready to hear it. "I'm going home for Christmas," she'd say, a pang in her voice. "Mom's doing her margaritas-and-gingerbread party again this year. I wish you were going to be there." In my conversations with Courtney, she helped me recognize how lucky I was that I'd been able to put time, energy, and money into getting better. "You know how many kids there are who don't have any resources—who can't even begin to start picking up the pieces?" she said.

"I know," I said. "I'm insanely fortunate."

"You are," she said. "But you still did the work. And I know it wasn't easy."

Ultimately, I found it was freeing to put it all to rest. I had maintained no contact with James, which felt like its own triumph in holding a boundary; I just hoped I'd never run into him on a New York City street. In therapy with Lauren, I parsed my anger toward Mr. Mason, unpacking how he had tricked and manipulated me. It wasn't just the violation. It was that he had exploited my most tender quality—my desire to lead, to please, to be kind. He had seen who I was at my core and used it against me. It was the worst kind of abuse I could imagine: taking me from me. But beyond the abuse, working with Lauren helped me begin to understand dynamics that ran much deeper than the pain of what had happened in the day-to-day. "If it's hysterical, it's historical," a friend told me once, and I tried to remember that when I found myself having a disproportionate reaction to something that had nothing to do with my trauma—particularly when it came to perceived abuses of power, no matter how minor. I still struggled to set boundaries, stretched myself too thin, and often put others' needs ahead of my own, but I was more forgiving with myself than I had been before.

I had thought I would be the model survivor, bringing my perpetrator to justice and earning another award for my exemplary leadership. I would leave no stone unturned in my quest to protect other women from being harmed by the same man who hurt me. But I had done all that I could, and the system had failed me. I had to stop fighting.

What mattered to me now was that I raise my children with different messages from the ones I'd internalized as a little girl. I wanted my daughters to know that their worth had nothing to do with whether they were valuable in the eyes of men; that they could, and should, question authority at every turn; and that with me as their parent, they could share any truth, no matter how tough it might feel in the moment. And I knew I had to model all of this in the way I lived my life.

I found, too, that I had become more attuned to my physical body than I'd ever been before, dialing in to the clues that presented themselves as I moved through the world. At a birthday party at a Chinese restaurant in Midtown, dozens of guests spilling into an industrial-size elevator, I suddenly realized that it was packed with people like a tin of sardines. As the elevator doors began to shut, I could feel the world closing in on me.

Thwack! I flung my handbag, a thin, envelope-style leather clutch, between the doors, like an assassin wielding a throwing star. There was a miserable grinding sound as the doors tried to close, which they now could not. Then the alarm bell began to sound.

"Amy," somebody behind me said, "why did you do that?"

I pushed past everyone and got out. "I'll take the next one," I said.

"They were all so inconvenienced by it," I said later to Olivia, who had become a trusted friend. "But for me it was an act of self-preservation."

"That's good," she said. "You're learning how to take up space—and not to judge yourself for it but to be kind with yourself instead."

"You taught me that," I said.

She was typically self-effacing. "All I did was sit in a room with you and hold your hand," she said. "It was you, with you, always." She was helping me let go of the idea of perfection, helping me redefine it. "You were always perfect, just as you are," she said. "You just have to keep remembering who you have always been—the essence of who you truly are."

THE FACT THAT THE school was sinking felt like a cosmic punch line; it would not have surprised me if a chasm had opened in the ground and swallowed it whole. Part of me did want to go back and see it one last time before they tore it

down, but another part of me was sure it would be too destabilizing. I had made it this far without returning to the scene
of the crime.

Then the flip slide: What if I went back, I saw it, and it
didn't align with my memories? Would that invalidate everything I had remembered? I still had days when I would try to
convince myself that somehow I had made the whole thing
up. It wasn't that I doubted myself; it was more that I wanted
an out, a way to just leave all of this behind and move on. I
wondered whether if I saw the school and even one small
detail was off, I'd begin to question the whole story. But also,
if the school no longer stood, that would mean I would never
have a chance to confirm that my memories were accurate.
The window for me to confront the past was closing—
literally and figuratively.

Maybe it would feel better for the school to not be there
anymore—to have it razed, as if nothing had ever happened
within those walls. I imagined the loop, the one I'd run so
many times through the park, with no school in the middle
of it, the block as open as the plains of Palo Duro Canyon.

You cannot go back. You have to go back. I let these two
contradictory truths coexist within me as I made my way out
of my apartment building to a coffee meeting with a young
woman who had just graduated from business school, a
friend of a friend who was looking for career advice. The moment I sat down, it was like looking at my reflection twenty
years ago: This young woman was bright, ambitious, and
nervous, just as I'd been at that age. She was new to New
York City, although her résumé was more impressive than
mine had ever been, and she talked a mile a minute in a
southern accent, the same way I once had.

"So now that you've graduated, what do you think you want to do?" I asked.

"Well, that's the thing—I have a couple options I'm pursuing," she said. "I'm trying to choose."

I was impressed. I had expected her to ask for my help in finding a job. "Do you think you want to live in New York City?" I asked.

"Yes, ma'am," she said. Reflexively I flinched.

"Did you look at investment banking or consulting programs?"

"No, ma'am," she said. I flinched again. "I want to do something more entrepreneurial."

"You might do a few things now that you realize you don't like," I said. "But that's good information for the future, too—so you can cross things off your list."

"Yes, ma'am," she said.

At the end of the meeting, she shook my hand graciously. "Thank you so much for your time," she said. "I appreciate it so much."

I paused for a long minute. "Can I share some advice with you that was given to me when I first moved to New York?"

"Of course," she said.

"Drop the 'Yes, ma'am,'" I said. "You're a woman with multiple degrees, varied job experience, and a great career ahead of you. You don't need to be so deferential."

"I'm sorry," she said. "It's how I was raised."

"It's how I was raised too," I said.

How could I explain to her that something so small could feel, to me, so loaded? To anyone back home, calling someone older or wiser than you "sir" or "ma'am" was simply a

sign of good manners. But to me now, the practice epito-
mized everything about the culture that had made me vulnerable to abuse as a child. A culture ruled by power
dynamics; a culture that demanded my obedience, silenced
my voice, and guarded my secrets; a culture that told me to
do what adults said, no matter what.

She thanked me for the advice and for my time. But I was
the one who had needed her, not the other way around. As I
walked home, I wondered: *Do I want to spend the rest of my
life being bothered by such a trivial figure of speech?* I wanted a
sturdy foundation of my own, so that little stuff like this
didn't make me, too, sink into the ground—pulling me into
the morass of all my old triggers.

The truth was that although I had changed so much,
there were still some things that remained unresolved. This
young woman had shown me both how far I'd come and
how far I still had to go.

AT HOME, JACK'S DOOR was shut; I knew he had his girlfriend over, but I didn't feel the urge to barge in. Before, I
had always seen my children as an extension of me; I loved
them so deeply and saw so much of myself in them that I
had placed the same expectations on them that I had placed
on myself, which were, in turn, the same expectations that
had been placed on me when I was a child. I had grown to
see my children as individuals, and I respected them in new
ways.

That meant not pacing in the hallway, arms crossed,
ready to greet them angrily if they came home one minute
past curfew. It also meant allowing them to direct their anger

toward me without taking it personally, understanding that it was a gift that they trusted me to hold it. They weren't slamming doors because I was failing as a parent; they were slamming doors because they were teenagers. And over time, when my kids came home at night, they would tell me more intimately about what was really going on in their lives—who was drinking at a party, whether the parents of the friend whose house they were going to were actually home or not, and whose restrictive behavior around food had their other friends concerned. "Before, you always believed the teacher or the babysitter instead of asking for my side of the story," Gigi said. "Now it feels like you come to me first to hear my side of the story." Instead of my seeing my kids as guilty until proven innocent, there was an inherent trust that had been built between us.

"You are so much more relaxed now than you used to be," Gracie told me. "Not, like, sit-by-the-pool relaxed, because that will never be you. But I feel like I can tell you anything." My edges had softened. Even my militance about the salt and pepper shakers being passed together and clockwise at a dinner table, which any southern belle could tell you was basic common decency, had lessened. The salt would be fine traveling around the table on its own.

IN MY BEDROOM, I was fumbling around on a top shelf of my closet looking for a sweater when out tumbled a blue leather-bound journal. I read the text on the cover: PLEASANT DREAMS. It was the diary I'd kept in the weeks after my first MDMA session. I'd long since abandoned it, and I had never had the courage to look back through it in the years since.

I opened the diary to the first page. "I lent a dress to the sweet girl, Claudia," I had written. "Being kind and doing things for others created a distraction from what was happening to me."

Claudia had been a dead end, just like everything else; I remembered Cate said that when Claudia spoke to the investigator, she barely remembered me. But something about it nagged at me. Idly, I wondered how her life had turned out. Was she still living in Amarillo?

I dug out all the files from the investigation I'd abandoned two years earlier. I had never read them in detail. I had been so raw, so powerless, and so out of control, when it was all first coming up, that I hadn't known if I was strong enough to face all the facts myself. Instead I had allowed Cate to be the intermediary, summarizing the findings for me. But now I knew that I could handle it.

There was a photo of Mr. Mason in the file. I studied the picture, taking it in. He looked the same, just older and more worn; in the picture, he was sitting in a metal folding chair with his wife, who had her arm around him. I pitied her. He had the same good-ol'-boy grin he'd had thirty years earlier. I set the photo aside and moved on to the reports from the investigators.

They'd spoken with so many people from back home and questioned them about their memories of Mr. Mason without using my name. As I read back through the reports, I found that, just as Cate had explained two years earlier, nobody seemed to have any particularly damning recollections of him, at least nothing that would hold up in court. It was just a bunch of stray threads—revelations that had felt explosive at the time but ended up leading nowhere. I felt discouraged and disheartened all over again. *How had I been the only one?*

I turned to the next file and found it was Claudia's. I opened the transcript of the conversation and started scanning it.

INVESTIGATOR: Is it correct that you were a student at Navarro Middle School in seventh and eighth grade?

CLAUDIA: That sounds about right.

INVESTIGATOR: That would have been 1988 to 1990?

CLAUDIA: I would have to go back and do the math.

She seemed standoffish in the transcript, but then again, so had many people when the investigators had called them. So much for southern hospitality. I wondered if there was anything to the fact that she couldn't remember when she'd been at Navarro. I knew from everything I had read about childhood trauma that it was common to struggle with the recall of traumatic memories. But it was probably nothing.

INVESTIGATOR: Do you recall any rumors of inappropriate behavior regarding teachers at school?

CLAUDIA: No.

INVESTIGATOR: What are your memories of school?

CLAUDIA: I had a normal adolescence. Middle school was horrible. Nothing in particular.

Middle school was horrible, but nothing about it was horrible in particular? Were these just standard recollections of teen angst, I wondered, or could it be something else?

INVESTIGATOR: Did you have Mr. Mason as a teacher?

CLAUDIA: I don't remember. Name doesn't sound familiar.

INVESTIGATOR: Do you remember any school dances?

CLAUDIA: No.

I continued scanning the document, annoyed that she remembered so little.

INVESTIGATOR: Do you remember someone giving you a dress?

CLAUDIA: I remember borrowing a dress from someone. Amy lent it to me. Amy something. My mom would remember the name.

Suddenly, I was riveted. Wasn't that funny? She didn't remember anything except that one object—the dress I had loaned her. Like Professor Bice with his teddy bear all those years earlier, even in the blurriest memory, something tangible had the power to cut through.

INVESTIGATOR: Were you friends with Amy?

CLAUDIA: Not really. Friendly acquaintances, not confidantes. We probably had classes together.

INVESTIGATOR: Why did she give you a dress?

CLAUDIA: I think my mother asked her parents for a dress. My family didn't have any money.

INVESTIGATOR: Do you remember thanking her?

CLAUDIA: Yes. I don't remember the verbiage. I remember how gracious she was.

I set down the page, overwhelmed. *She remembered me because of the dress.* The memory was incredibly important to me, crystal clear in my mind. Of course Cate couldn't have known how significant the dress was to me. But in my memory, the dress and Claudia and Mr. Mason were all linked in some mysterious way I couldn't explain.

I knew enough to know that the magic of the medicine was its ability to cut through the clutter of the mind to a place of essential truth. So why was it that the first thing I wrote after the MDMA had unlocked these memories was about Claudia—not about the abuse, or the teacher, but about her?

There had to be something there. I didn't know what, but I knew that in the memory of Claudia, there was a thorn, a thing as yet unresolved within me—the same way that there had been something unresolved in that young woman's obedient voice, saying "Yes, ma'am." I felt a flicker of familiarity, the filament of myself that had been in her and that was also in Claudia—the reflection of how it felt to be subordinated. It was all connected.

The investigator had included Claudia's full name in the report, since she had married and taken her husband's name.

I typed it into my keyboard. Why had it taken me so long to do this?

In a matter of seconds, I was staring at her picture on my screen. She had the same smile and the same eyes. She was married to a lawyer and lived a few hours east of Amarillo. A moment later, I had her phone number.

"Hi Claudia," I texted. "This is Amy from middle school. I know, such a long time ago. Hope you don't mind that I looked you up. I'm trying to reconstruct some memories from those years and wondered if you might be open to chatting with me. I'll be in your area soon if you'd be open to a coffee. It would be so nice to reconnect."

She wrote back. "I would be happy to have coffee if time allows," she said. "Someone reached out to me a bit ago. As I explained to them, I have no memory of many of the people involved. But if I can assist, I will. Let me know when you are in town."

I looked up to find John standing in the doorway, where I had all the papers spread out before me. My relationship with John had always been my greatest source of strength, but we had become closer than I could have imagined when I walked down the aisle all those years ago. It wasn't lost on me that he had done "the work" of dissolving his own shame with the help of MDMA before I had. It was only because I trusted him so emphatically that I had been willing to do my own. Through my coming to know myself more deeply, our connection had deepened too. Even during the darkest nights, when I fell asleep crying on the closet floor, I would wake up to find he had gotten up to cover me with a blanket. He was steadfast, a wise owl whose love for me had never faltered.

"What are you working on?" he asked.

"I think I have to go back," I said. It was the first time I had said the words out loud, and the sound of them surprised me. But it was time. I had to excavate my own foundation. This was the last piece of the puzzle.

"John," I said, "I think I have to go home."

11. HOMECOMING

The landscape of Amarillo was flatter than I remembered, even though it had been only a few years since I'd been home. We descended into the airport over agricultural plots cut into intricate geometric shapes. The tallest thing on the horizon was a field of futuristic white wind turbines, taking advantage of the open space. The expanse of the high plains was vast and arid, miles of visibility in every direction.

My mom was waiting outside the airport wearing jeans, a navy blue cardigan with a sash around her waist, and comfortable flats. She hugged me, and when I moved to let go, she hugged me even tighter. "I am just so happy that you're home," she said. "Now what do you want to do? Do you want to go to Eat-Rite and grab an avocado sprout sandwich? Or should we go get barbecue? Do you want to go home first and put your bags down? We can always do Taco Villa. Is there anybody you think you want to go see? Or you want to go down to the office? I'd love to show you some of the renovations. I know your dad is dying for you to see the new store on the interstate—we're all so proud of it. Oh, I'm just so happy you're home!"

"I'm happy to be home, too," I said. Part of me meant it, but part of me was already putting on my armor for what I'd come here to do.

"You know, you always talk about all the terrible things that happened here, and I know they did," my mom said. We were driving on the highway, back toward the neighborhood where I was raised, where my parents still lived. "But I so want you to remember all of the wonderful memories we made here, too. It wasn't all bad, right?"

"Of course it wasn't," I said. "Part of what makes this so hard is that I have so many fond memories of life here and how you raised me."

It was true that I had forgotten how beautiful Amarillo was. As we crossed into the neighborhood where I'd grown up, the road beneath us turned to redbrick, which was always how I knew that I was almost home. The light grew golden as it filtered through the leaves of the trees overhead. It was spring, and everything was in bloom: To exit the barren plains with so little vegetation and arrive in a verdant oasis with so many trees, stately colonial homes, and manicured lawns—the magic never wore off.

My parents' house was just as I had left it—even the garage door code was the same. They had moved when I was in high school, to a bigger house than the one on Carter

Street where I'd spent my childhood, since our family had grown, and they had stayed there in the thirty years since. All the details were familiar: The rustic formal living room, with its dark wood interiors. Rows of majolica plates in the kitchen, the same ones my mom had spent years scouring antiques stores to find, with me in tow. Monogrammed hand towels with scalloped edges and potpourri in the powder room. My father materialized, greeting me with a big hug.

"I'm glad you're here," he said. "I wish you were staying longer so you could come out to the ranch." He had driven from the family ranch, an hour outside of town, to see me, even though it was the middle of the cattle-branding season, which happened twice a year. Over several days, they rounded up all the cattle, including the new calves that had been born in the spring, to be branded and inoculated. But beyond its function, this endeavor was a ceremonial undertaking that united the ranch hands, cowboys from neighboring ranches, and our extended family around feasts of calf fries, chicken-fried steak, and mashed potatoes. It marked the changing of the season, and I knew it was a point of pride for my dad. "I know you haven't been able to come down with the kids to see it, but it really is so special," he said as we settled in the living room, my mom busying herself in the kitchen. "You get up at the crack of dawn with these cowboys, all working for a common goal."

I checked the time. My flight had landed around lunch so I could go to the school right as the students were dismissed; my brother Andrew's wife, Dottie, would be taking me, since she knew the principal. Dottie was meant to arrive any minute. There was no time to waste. After all, the school was sinking.

"It feels so good to be out in nature," my father was saying. "It's part of why I love living here so much. Seeing the light come up over the ridge at the break of dawn is just something you have to experience."

"I'm sorry to take you away from it," I said. "It means a lot that you came in to be with me."

"Well, I know it's hard for you to get home," he said.

"So are you going back tomorrow?"

"Yes, I'll leave around five A.M. to drive back, maybe earlier," he said. "We gotta get up early for the coyote hunt."

"Coyote hunt?" I asked.

"They keep multiplying," he said. "They're nasty animals. If we don't kill them, they'll come after the calves. They only prey on the young." I listened. "All you have to do is protect the cattle until they're big enough, and then they'll be fine—the coyotes won't come after them once they're grown. The key is to keep them safe while they're little."

"I guess it's the cattle or the coyotes," I said.

My father looked pensive. "Well, the coyotes can't help it. It's a law of nature. It's just what they do. And it's our job to make sure they don't."

DOTTIE'S SUV WAS IDLING in the driveway as I stepped outside into the cool afternoon. She was a statuesque blond with a warm demeanor who'd met my brother Andrew in college. Their daughter, my niece, was now a student at Navarro, which was how my mom had gotten wind of the school sinking in the first place.

"Did you know the principal was in your grade?" Dottie said.

"I played basketball against her in middle school," I said. "But we went to different high schools."

"Small world," Dottie said.

"Everybody knows everybody here."

"I didn't tell her anything," Dottie said. "About what happened to you, I mean. I just told her that you were back in town and wanted to see the school again. She was so nice about it."

"Thank you for organizing this for me."

"I got you," Dottie said. Suddenly it felt like we were on a mission, committing some kind of espionage, although to what end I didn't yet know. But I was grateful she was on my team.

As we rounded the corner to the school, I saw a long line of cars snaking around the block as parents waited to pick up their kids, who streamed out of every door, jostling backpacks and saying their goodbyes; the energy was frenetic, busy as a beehive. "Give it a minute," Dottie said. "It empties out fast." We circled the block, and by the time we came back around, it was a ghost town, with hardly anyone in sight. Emptied of students, the school suddenly reminded me of my clearest memories of it—the way it had felt once class was out for the day and I was alone, staying late after school. I studied an elm tree. *Was that tree always there?* I wondered. I wasn't sure. Scanning the block opposite the school, I could still remember the names of the families who had lived in each house, their kids, with whom I'd grown up.

We parked on the street and walked through the front door, past a few kids straggling out. As I entered the school, I felt nothing. I had prepared for how this would go and had anticipated a swell of emotion, but instead I was robotic. My body felt stiff, like I was wearing a straitjacket.

The hallways were the same—extra wide, with oversize sand-colored tiles. I could picture the way my red Keds would look against the floor as a seventh grader; how strange and surreal that now, thirty years later, I was back. It was like being in a time warp. The principal greeted us outside her office, and I remembered her as soon as I saw her face. "School is out, so you're free to roam," she laughed. "Make yourself comfortable! Enjoy the trip down memory lane! As you can see, not much has changed."

I made small talk, but I barely knew what I was saying; I was focused on the glare beneath my feet, the way the light bounced off the polished linoleum. As I had remembered, all the doors swung out, into the hallway. A long line of portraits of previous principals, all of them male, hung in neat rows in fancy frames; you could see the passage of time, over the decades, from the men's haircuts and the shape of their eyeglasses.

"I'll let you do your thing," Dottie said. She motioned to the lobby, where she would wait. "Let me know if you need me." I nodded and set off down the hallway on my own.

So little had changed. Every detail was the same. The tiles at the bottom of the stairway were rounded; that was important to me for some reason. The color of the stone on the walls was such a specific neutral: an off-white, paler than cream and warmer than gray. The doors to all the classrooms had small windows cut into them, big enough to peek through, although most teachers had covered theirs with fabric. I stopped, staring at the windows. That had also been a critical detail, one I had told Olivia I remembered. Now that I had seen that I was right, I could not invalidate my memory. In the long hallway leading to the gym, I looked for the photo of myself, the winner of the award that Bess Taylor had given me, which I'd been told would hang here for generations to come, but it was nowhere to be found. A betrayal, but hardly the worst one that had happened at that school.

In so many different corners of the building, the light came through in specific ways, at angles and in hues I remembered so vividly. I had thought about that light every day, I realized suddenly, with a kind of fondness; it was like the light was my friend. I had never thought to wonder why. I did not think that way about my high school or my grade school. It was this place that had lodged in my memory for over thirty years. Now that I was back, it was as familiar as if I had never left. I had been walking these halls for a long time.

I opened the door to the auditorium, off the main hallway. I could still feel the hardness of the wooden chairs that I'd sat in so many times; I reached my hand out and felt the contour of the seat, thin and stiff. That was the stage on which I'd stood to receive that award, where I'd looked out to see the tears in my father's eyes. It felt smaller now than it had back then, but only because I had been so little.

In the hallway, I stopped in front of the bathroom. The door had been removed; I could still see the hinges, painted over on the side, where it had previously been attached. Now it was laid out such that there was a partition separating the bathroom from the hallway that you walked around, to the left, after passing through the doorframe; in this way, the sinks and stalls were shielded from the hallway without needing a door. This was the first place that had come back to me in my first MDMA session, the physical location that was most charged. I took a deep breath and entered.

Everything had been redone, even the window, which had previously had the handle I remembered so well. The floor was clean and speckled. The sinks were made of plastic now, not porcelain. Everything was crisp and new, rubberized and modernized. It was sterile and banal. The last time I had visited that bathroom, it was in my memory, in my third session, and I had fantasized about destroying it. Now I saw that in the years since my body had been in the space, it actually had been torn down and rebuilt. In some ways this was a gift; I was not sure I could have handled the sight of it if I had walked in and it had looked exactly the same. The proportions of the room were identical, and the window was where I had remembered it, but the contents of the room were different now. Yet it still felt familiar, like I'd never left.

I looked back at the doorframe, now blocked by that interior partition. I had stared at the door that had stood there with such intensity, wishing that there were a way out, and now the door was gone. I had never liked being in public bathrooms. Now I knew why.

In the gymnasium, I found that the wooden bleachers had been replaced with metal ones. The floor was still warped, just as it had been when I'd played volleyball there. As I passed under the basketball hoop, I suddenly remembered Mr. Mason doing a vertical jump contest. He was being silly, leaping off the ground to touch the wall. He had always stood by the double doors that led to the locker room as I came in from class to get ready, so I'd have to pass by him.

The locker room, too, had been remodeled. The lockers were now candy-apple green and shiny, the floors done in bland gray wash. Nothing but the four walls was the same.

I walked past the door to the cafeteria but did not go inside. I had a memory in that cafeteria that had always stuck with me; I had been sitting at the table with friends, eating a peanut butter and honey sandwich, and Mr. Mason had leaned in over me. I stared down at the rounded lips of the brown trays pushed together on the table in front of me. "What are you all having for lunch?" he asked. I had to remind myself that I was surrounded by people. *There are lots of us here. He cannot get me. I am safe.* When he exited the cafeteria, I exhaled heavily. Now I took a similar breath, a sigh of relief that I was no longer twelve and he was no longer there.

I found that the room where I remembered him chasing me around the desk was now a Spanish classroom with colorful flags and conversational phrases pasted up on the walls. Through the shades, the light appeared in bars along the floor.

Out in the hallway, there were signs everywhere, expressions of inspirational uplift. *Never settle for less than your best! Just be you!* On one wall, there was a display of student art, made with cut-out pieces of construction paper and glitter glue. Each had a student's name and a statement.

I am creative.
I am fun.
I am somebody.

Had I made one of those collages as a little girl? I could not remember. What would mine have said?

I am a leader.
I am an athlete.
I am kind.
I am good at keeping secrets.

I turned and looked down the hallway, which was streaked with sunlight. The way it sliced through the windows at this time of day, in this season, was etched into my memory; part of the hallway was dim, and the other part was bright. I had pictured it so many times, this exact place—me, walking down it alone.

I stood there for a long moment, taking it in.

Then, once I was finally ready, I walked out of the shadows and into the light.

DOTTIE AND I DROVE the short distance I knew so well to the house on Carter Street. Getting out in front of the old house, the one where I'd lived until high school, I saw that the old cherry tree where I'd collected ladybugs as a little girl was gone.

Dottie looked over at me. "Didn't you guys have rabbits growing up?"

"Yes," I said. "How did you know that?"

"Your brother told me about them," she said. "You all came home from a vacation, and there was white fur all over the backyard. And you asked, 'Did it snow?' The dog had gotten to them, right?"

I winced. "It was one of those moments in my life when my parents just had no idea what to do," I said. "Now I feel bad for them. In the moment, I remember them running around to clean it up as if nothing had happened. But we all knew the rabbits had been eaten by the dog. We never spoke about it." There were a lot of things that just weren't talked about—not out of insensitivity but more to insulate the kids from adult realities.

We knocked on the door, and the current owners, a kind couple who were friendly with my family, let us in. It was a reminder of how people went out of their way for one another in a place like Amarillo—casserole culture at its finest.

The house still felt like home. The walk down the hallway to what had been my bedroom was so familiar; it had been down this hallway that I'd crept when I would go for runs on the weekend. The wooden blinds covering the windows were still the same, the ones I'd peeked through to see Claudia coming up the driveway with the dress in the plastic dry-cleaning bag. So was the cabinetry in the closet, with the handles cut into the drawers that I would use as footholds to climb up onto the highest shelf and hide. Even though my old room was now filled with exercise equipment and had been painted over, that safety that I'd felt there in the corner of the house endured.

In my parents' bedroom there was the archway that I used to run under, practicing my volleyball vertical jump. It had seemed like I would never reach it. Now my fingertips grazed it easily as I passed through to the next room. Slowly I wandered the house like a tourist exploring a museum, pausing before a window as if it were a great work of art. There was the skylight in my mom's bathroom where she used to sit to put her makeup on because there was so much natural light. There was the hard Mexican-tile floor that we used to ride our big-wheel bikes on. There, in my old bathroom, was the long counter with the sink at the end where I burned myself with a curling iron the first time I tried to curl my hair.

There were so many memories, so many of them lovely. I hadn't been placating my mom when I told her that I had beautiful memories here. I did.

Things had not been perfect. There had been pain, secrecy, and shame. I had suffered in silence.

And yet, and yet, and yet.

I had always loved the sunsets best in Amarillo when there was dust in the air, because it made the light even more beautiful—orange and diffuse, a tangerine dream. Maybe, I thought, my childhood was like that. The dust clouds made everything more special.

Everything that had happened here was a part of me. It was what made me who I was.

I could not run from that either. I had to run toward it.

SLEEPING IN MY PARENTS' house that night, everything was the same: the sound of the air conditioner, the way I fumbled for the switch on the cord of the lamp, the shade that didn't fully cover the window, so you could tell it was morning when the light peeked in. I did not hear my father leave to head back to the ranch, but I could smell the coffee that my mother made every morning, even though she knew I never drank caffeine; she always aimed to please, so she made it anyway, just in case my morning ritual had changed.

I woke up with a craving I hadn't had in thirty years: for a cherry glazed doughnut. With my mom, I picked one up from the drive-through and ate it hot. It tasted like children's cough syrup, and I loved it. Later we picked up an order from Taco Villa to bring to Claudia. Maybe, I thought, it would remind her of home.

"I can't tell you how much it means to me that you came home," my mom said as the landscape streaked past us. "It has truly healed me."

I squeezed her hand. "Me too," I said.

Before I left town, we pulled off the highway to see the new convenience store, which she and my dad had wanted me to see. It had a burnt-red roof and white brick façade, and it was fancier than I had expected. Walking in was like entering a Las Vegas casino. There were so many brightly colored displays, I was in sensory overload. The brands had multiplied. The aisles were wider. Everything was shinier. To contrast it with the stores I remembered, the stores of my youth, was an object lesson in the changing appetites of the American consumer. Before, I'd thought of the store as something that was for staples, where all you had was a choice between Fritos and Doritos. Now the store had everything a person could ever want, things a person didn't even know they wanted until they saw them: prepared foods, dry goods, kitschy home décor, branded apparel, and fountains for sodas and Slush Puppies in eight flavors, from Jolly Rancher watermelon to Dr Pepper, the local favorite. In one corner was a barbecue station, named after my father, where the line to order stretched halfway back through the store. Through a corridor was a recreation room for truckers, with overstuffed recliners; out the window was an expansive truck stop. It was like a city of its own, a place where people could get everything they might need, just as they had at the stores when I was little.

In my imagination, Amarillo was a place time had forgotten. In my least generous moments, I had characterized this whole town as provincial, trapped in the past. That was why I'd never wanted to come back. But so much had changed here, hadn't it?

"Isn't this amazing?" my mom said, looking around with

wonder. She was so proud. I thought of my grandmother Novie, who had built this business all those years ago. Novie, who had modeled strength for me before I knew how much strength I'd need.

"Yes," I said, meaning it, "it is."

Nothing had changed, but everything had changed. The same was true of me.

It was there, in a store like that one, that I had internalized the lesson that things were better when they were convenient. But now I was an adult, and I could see a different truth.

Yes, there was a place for convenience. But not everything needed to sit tidily on a shelf. Some things were messy, difficult, or impossible to contain. Some things defied easy categorization. What happened to me when I was a girl was all of those things. It didn't fit neatly in a box. But I had to accept it—no matter how inconvenient it was.

ON THE INTERSTATE, THE billboards alternated between antiabortion campaigns and ads for adult video stores. The old me would have relished pointing out the hypocrisy, but today I let it go.

"So what was it like?" my mom asked. "Coming home."

"You know what?" I said. "It was just as I remembered it."

12. CARDS

The colors changed as I pulled into the town where Claudia lived, the views now greener than the orange landscape of Amarillo, parking on the street outside the coffee shop where we had arranged to meet.

Inside, I scanned the café, looking for her, but I had arrived early. My heart was racing. I was anxious. It was kind of Claudia to meet with me, someone she hadn't seen in thirty years. I locked in on a small bistro table in a corner where I knew we would be able to talk privately, then stepped into the bathroom to compose myself.

I looked at my reflection in the mirror. *You've got this.* But did I? In my session with Lauren a few days earlier, we had talked about what to expect going into this meeting. "You don't need anything out of this other than to show yourself compassion," Lauren had reminded me. Would this meeting be just another dead end? I couldn't say. But I'd learned during my own recovery journey that discussing my trauma could deeply affect Claudia, and I wanted to take care in how I broached the topic. I knew so little about where she'd been in her life, and where she was now. I feared she'd suffered the same way I had. If so, much had already been taken from her; I didn't want to ask for anything more. Moreover, I didn't need her to corroborate my memories or to volunteer her own story. But I couldn't help but harbor hope that my story might shake something loose in her. Maybe she'd feel comfortable telling me things that she wouldn't have felt comfortable saying to a stranger on the phone when the investigator had called. I wanted to be able to ask her the questions that had rolled around in my mind ever since my first session. *Did it happen to you, too? Do you remember things that I don't? Why are you such an important part of my memories?*

Exiting the bathroom, I took a seat at the table and waited. A moment later, Claudia arrived. I watched as she came through the door, and time seemed to slow down. Her kind eyes were the same, though her hair was longer. She was dressed casually in a tennis skirt, a denim jacket, and a baseball cap. I stretched my arms out to give her a hug and she reciprocated, although it was awkward; even in middle school, we hadn't known each other that well. "Thank you so much for coming to see me," I said. "I know it must have seemed so out of the blue." I pulled out the bag of Taco Villa, and she gasped at the sight of it.

"This was my favorite!" she said.

"My mom would always remind me to open the hot sauce carefully," I said. "Otherwise it'll pop open and stain your shirt."

She laughed. "Oh, I remember well," she said.

We waited for our drinks at the counter, fidgeting nervously and making small talk like strangers on a blind date. "I'm so grateful to you for taking the time," I said. "I know it's not easy to get away from work and family."

"My kids keep me busy," she said. She pulled out her phone and showed me pictures of them in their athletic uniforms. "We're always traveling for soccer tournaments."

"I have one who plays soccer too," I said. "Four kids, and each plays a different sport—so we're in the same boat. There's never any downtime. It's such a busy phase of our lives—fun, but busy." I felt like I was dancing around the subject. Surely she was wondering: *What does this woman want from me?*

Finally, once our coffees were ready, we began to speak, my voice shaking. "You're probably wondering why I came to see you," I said. "I've been processing some things that happened to me when we were in middle school."

"Somebody called me a while back," she said. "I told them I don't remember anything about middle school. It was an awful time in my life."

"Really?" I said. "I'm so sorry to hear that."

"I just don't remember much," she said. She seemed tense—not unfriendly but guarded. Was that because she was protecting a secret? Or was it because I was, to her, a random woman who had hired an investigator to call her up and ask her about what had been a difficult time in her life—and then I'd come to talk to her myself, after thirty years? It was impossible to know. The entire situation, I understood, was bizarre. Maybe she thought I was crazy.

"Please don't worry—I don't need you to remember anything," I said. "I came here because I was hoping to tell you my story, of how I remembered some things about middle school. Is it all right if I share that with you?"

She nodded. "Of course," she said.

"I've been processing the memories of my childhood," I said. "Sometimes it feels like a puzzle that I'm trying to assemble—not just of what I remember but why I remember what I do."

"Memory is a funny thing," Claudia said slowly. "I mean, our minds are capable of coming up with so many things, aren't they? You can't really trust your memories."

For a moment, I was taken aback. Was she saying that she didn't believe me before I'd even told her what happened? Was she talking about her own memory or mine?

"Do you remember Mr. Mason?" I asked. "He was one of the teachers at Navarro."

She shook her head. "Like I told your lawyers, or whoever they were, I don't remember anything from that time." She hesitated. "My home life really wasn't great. We moved around a lot. And also the girls in that grade were so mean." Then she backpedaled. "I don't hold it against them. That's just a rough time in life in general."

"I'm sorry to hear that," I said again. "It's funny—I have such distinct memories of you. You being around Mr. Mason. Several of our interactions during middle school. In all my memories, you're a constant. Although we weren't close friends, I felt connected to you. I remember looking in your eyes and feeling like we recognized something in each other."

She shifted in her seat, looking uncomfortable. "The reason all this has come up for me," I said, "is because I was abused by Mr. Mason beginning in the seventh grade." Over time, it had become so much easier for me to talk about what I'd experienced once I realized *why* I was talking about it. Saying it out loud was an active undoing of the self-betrayal of having denied it for so long. It was a gesture of unconditional love toward myself.

I had grown accustomed to a range of reactions—people tearing up, gasping, or flinching. Sometimes they reached for my hand and held it. But they always leaned in. Claudia was the first person I had ever shared this with who leaned back, as if trying to get away from me. I felt her energy shift, a stiffening in her body. She bit her lip and didn't blink.

Was she setting a nonverbal boundary with me, I wondered—or was she tightening up because there was something she, too, couldn't face?

"It's taken a lot for me to be honest with myself about what happened," I said. "But I've kept a journal for the last several years, and you were the first thing I wrote about in the journal—this memory I have, of lending you a dress. So I knew I had to find you. I had to tell you that, I guess."

She said nothing. She looked down at the floor. I had to fill the silence. "So again, I'm just grateful to you for coming to meet me," I said as I leaned in farther. "And I promise I don't need anything from you."

But I knew in my heart that wasn't the truth. I had hoped for catharsis. I had hoped she would crumble and tell me it had happened to her too. We would ride off into the sunset together, having solved the mystery. Or I had hoped that she would confidently tell me that nothing happened but that she was sorry for my pain. I would believe her, know from the truth in her eyes that he had not victimized her too. We would hug, and I would go back to New York and move on with my life, having made peace with the fact that my story alone was enough, with no loose ends still waiting to be tied up.

Instead, she was giving me nothing.

I felt tears streaming down my cheeks.

Claudia's face was stoic.

Then, finally, she spoke.

"I remember you," she said. Her voice cracked, and the energy shifted again. "I remember that you were kind to me." Her eyes were red. "You were the only person who was kind to me, Amy."

"Really?" I said. I used the napkin from the coffee I hadn't touched to wipe my eyes.

"Yes," she said. "You loaned me a dress for the dance."

"The floral one," I said, motioning with my hands. "The one with puffy sleeves."

"Yes," she said. "My family was so poor. I think maybe my mom asked your dad if I could borrow a dress, or maybe you and I talked about it—I don't know. But you gave it to me. And I have thought about you and that gesture so many times over the years." She began to cry. "Not because you gave me the dress but because you didn't tell anyone. You didn't embarrass me. You could have told everyone, but you didn't. You kept it a secret so I wouldn't be more humiliated than I already was."

We were both weeping now, gathered around this little table. "I remember just really wanting to be kind," I said. "Even when Bess brought me up on stage that day, it was like—I didn't understand why I was being given an award for being kind. Weren't we all supposed to be kind? I would never have told anyone you borrowed my dress. That wasn't why I lent it to you. I just wanted to help you. I knew—

I knew things were bad for you in some way. And they were bad for me too, just in a different way. Maybe that's why I felt connected to you."

"I'm just so sorry, Amy," she cried. "I wish that I could help you. But at that age, you're so focused on yourself. All I thought about was myself. I didn't notice that there was something going on with you. I wish I had. But I had no idea. I'm just so sad that I can't help you—that I don't remember anything, when such a horrible thing was happening to you." She wiped her eyes. "And when they called me to ask me about it, I just—I searched my memory, I did, because I wanted to help you, but I just couldn't. I couldn't remember anything."

I sat there, processing, realizing that I had misread her reticence. Her body language hadn't been because she was ashamed to share what had happened to her. She was ashamed because she wanted to help me, but she could not.

But then why had the medicine brought me back to her? Why was she the first thing I had written about in my PLEASANT DREAMS journal? Why had I been unable to get her out of my head all these years?

Interlocking pieces snapped into place. And once again, I saw it all so clearly.

What if I hadn't given Claudia the dress because she was being abused?

What if I had given Claudia the dress because that was who I was?

What had Olivia said in my first meeting with her? She called it rebecoming. "You have always been you," she said. "You just have to remember who you were." This was what I'd been meant to learn.

There was an essential me that no abuse could ever harm. The me before I felt that I had to be perfect. The me before I felt shame. The me that wanted to be kind, not as a distraction from what was happening to me but simply because it was the purest expression of love I knew. All of that was always within me. *That* was what I had to remember.

CLAUDIA AND I TALKED for a while longer in the coffee shop, wiping our tears away. We hugged goodbye; then she was gone. I sat for a moment, collecting my thoughts, before I stood up to go.

But when I did, I saw there was something still on the table—Claudia's sunglasses.

"Oh, Claudia—" I called, but I could see through the window that she was already in her car, reversing out of the parking lot. I texted her that she had left her glasses behind and asked the barista to hang on to them until she could come back.

But as I made my way out of town, I found myself thinking about it.

Wasn't that funny? How easy it was to miss something, even when it was right in front of you.

BACK IN NEW YORK, I continued to process my trip home. Being back in the school had shaken me; the enormity of what I'd endured was a lot to process. Yet I'd also felt validated by the fact that so much had looked the same as it had in my memory. "From the windows in the classroom doors to the taste of the cherry glazed doughnut, it was exactly as I had remembered it," I said to John. "If I ever try to doubt myself again, remind me of that." Maybe, I thought, this had been just what I needed to move on with my life.

A couple weeks later, I returned to Texas, traveling to Austin to see Rachel, Courtney, and a group of our closest friends for a long-planned girls' trip. A month before, I had decided to include Lizzie too; I felt the need to be close to my sister.

The main draw for the weekend was a country music concert—perhaps the only thing that could incentivize this group of busy mothers to align their schedules. We all stayed in the same hotel, Lizzie bounding into my room with armfuls of flowing cotton dresses, chunky embossed Western belts, and turquoise jewelry, asking for help choosing her outfit. It reminded me of the way my daughters got dressed—clothes strewn all over the room, the anticipation of the evening to come. Getting ready was half the fun, anyway: hair, makeup, pregaming with country music blasting from a speaker. In a jean skirt and boots, I felt like a true Texan again. It was liberating to be back as a woman who knew who she was, instead of as a girl who wanted her body to be invisible. But more than anything, I was grateful to spend time with my sister. As time had healed the space between us, I could see that I had resented Lizzie for her lightness, when I had carried such a heavy burden. Now I was starting to share in that lightness.

At the show, we drank Texas ranch waters and sang along to every word, huddled in a little group, as if we were the only ones there. Our children would have been mortified, but I felt like a teenager myself.

I told Rachel and Courtney about my time at home and

about the meeting with Claudia. "I'm sure it made your family so happy to have you back," Rachel said. "There are so many people in that town who love you."

"I can't believe you went to see her," Courtney said. "I spent hours trying to find her online!" I smiled—it was classic Courtney, forever the sleuth on my team. But I had gotten the resolution I needed, and it was good to put it down once and for all. I flew back to New York feeling that, in some small way, I had made my peace with Texas. After all, it had always been home.

In my session with Lauren after I got back, she presented me with that same deck of animal cards I'd used to pull the earthworm two years earlier. "The symbolism of the earthworm ended up working out well for me," I said. "But I'd love to draw an animal that lives above the ground this time."

Lauren smiled. "Let's see."

She fanned out the cards before me. Just as I had two years earlier, I grazed my fingers along several cards, finally selecting one and tugging it out of the deck. I turned it over. It was a whale.

Lauren paused. "The whale is the ultimate wise and knowing feminine card," she said. "It symbolizes truth and grace." She looked up at me. "A testament to all the work you've put in."

"I know this will be an ongoing journey," I said. "Emotionally, there will always be things that come up—which is good. It's a part of the process. But I feel like, after seeing Claudia, I can finally move forward. This obsession with trying to get answers, documenting everything, making it all concrete—it doesn't work that way." For so long I had believed that I could tie up what happened with a bow, making it as neat and convenient as the goods on the shelves at a Toot'n Totum. But recovery was an ocean, and I was learning how to swim.

NOT LONG AFTER, I was home after getting the kids to school when John came into the room, dressed for an early meeting. "I thought you should see this," he said. There was a strange expression on his face, and I could see that he had a postcard in his hand. He held it gingerly, as if delivering something that was on fire. "It must have just come in the mail," he said. "I'm glad I found it."

I took the postcard. On the front was a vintage black-and-white photo of two children playing together. When I turned it over, I saw there was a message, beautifully written in cursive in navy blue ink.

"I don't understand why I was given an award for being kind to someone. I mean, isn't that what you are supposed to do?" —Amy, circa 7th grade

My address was written in black ink. Then, in small letters, there was one more line at the very bottom of the postcard—also written in black, and upside down.

I rotated the postcard so I could read it. The upside-down message was scrawled as if added last-minute, tacked on while the sender was writing the address.

It read:

I didn't have it in me to tell you the truth.

13. ANSWERS

I stared at the postcard. "John," I said. I could hear my voice quavering. "What is this? Where did this come from?" I turned it over, then back over again. "Claudia," I said. "The only person this could be from is Claudia."

I felt my body tightening up. That familiar bloodhound in me that had spent all those months on the trail of something, desperate for clues, returned. "Where's the postmark?" I checked; it was stamped in New York City. "John, if there's a New York postmark on it, does that mean that it was initially sent in New York or just processed in New York?"

"I'm not sure," he said softly. He could see me spiraling.

"It has to be from her," I said. "Who else could have sent it?"

I studied it. The postmark, the mix of blue and black ink, the cursive handwriting with its elegant loops. There was a tiny red heart drawn after the postscript—"I didn't have it in me to tell you the truth"—like a bit of affection, a girlish softening of the grim admission. The stamp, too, was a picture of a heart. I felt the strangest mix of emotions surging through my body: relief, grief, pure adrenaline. It was what I had always wanted, wasn't it? To be validated—to be vindicated—to know that I wasn't alone. All I had needed was one other person to come out of the woodwork to affirm what I'd experienced, and I would feel like I could trust myself. That was why I'd spent so much time on the investigation in the first place. Now I had an ally to hold Mason accountable for what he'd done.

A perfect ending. Here it was. Right?

I traced my fingers over the cursive letters. It *was* from Claudia, right? Then I looked again. It wasn't from Rachel, was it? Her handwriting was similar, and I could remember her writing notes with little hearts that looked the same. She had been in New York the week before. But no—why would she send me an unsigned postcard with a mysterious upside-down message? That made no sense. Or could it be from Bess Taylor? But we had barely spoken in the last two years—why would she have only just sent it now?

Who else knew? How many other people were there to whom I'd told that story or with whom I'd used some version of that same language? At this point, there were many. Could somebody be toying with me? Was this some sort of cruel joke? Or someone else with whom I'd shared my story who hadn't been ready to tell me theirs? But sending me such a strange note—to what end?

. . .

I SPENT A WEEK spinning out, trying to summon the courage to text Claudia, drafting and redrafting the message in hopes of conveying the right tone. A part of me hoped that she would reach out to make sure that I'd gotten it; then I would know it was from her and put my doubts to rest. The more I thought about it, the more cryptic it all seemed—saying nothing at the café, then sending me a postcard? The behavior was so strange. Lauren and I talked about whether I should say something to her.

"I have so many questions," I said. "But am I dragging her back into something that's too difficult for her to face?"

"How would it make you feel if the roles were reversed?" Lauren asked.

"I would want to know the truth," I said. "I would want to talk about it. But I don't know if she's ready to break through her glass case. Did I shatter it for her?"

"You have to trust your instincts on this," she said.

Finally I sent her a text.

> Thank you for your courage.
> I see you.
> I understand you.
> I am here for you.

A week passed with no response. I tried to stay busy, using every trick I'd learned over the last few years to occupy myself. Walking in the park. Meditating. Long baths. Prayer. Dark chocolate. And an occasional sleeping pill. Nothing worked. I checked my phone every two seconds. Finally I snapped and wrote to her again.

I think about you every day and so hope I can hold
your hand.

Four days later, she responded.

Thank you. All is well. Best to you.

I stared at my phone screen. *Huh?* How was I supposed
to interpret that? Was she processing on her own? Did she
have resources to help her work through it? Should I leave
her alone? But if she had wanted me to leave her alone, why
had she sent me the postcard? And if it wasn't her, who was
it? I wrote again.

Claudia, I just wanted to see if you might be up for
talking about the postcard? I will get on a plane any
day this week and come down to support you. I've
cried so much in the last few weeks hoping I didn't
open up too many difficult memories for you, and in
knowing that it wasn't just me.

She responded quickly.

What postcard?

I looked at the screen, dumbfounded. *What?* I typed out
my reply.

I was sent an unsigned postcard two weeks ago that
said, "I didn't have it in me to tell you the truth." It
also had a quote we talked about. I assumed you remembered things from the past. I have been trying to

put the pieces together. I hope it didn't come off as weird when I thanked you for your courage. I thought you wanted to share with me and I was so grateful. Appreciate hearing from you. I am even more confused. This has been hard.

She responded.

I am sorry. But it was not me.

I set my phone down. Hope, crashing and burning once again.

"HERE'S WHAT WE'RE GONNA do," Courtney said. We were on the phone; I had just finished telling her the latest wrinkle in the postcard saga. "We're going to get somebody to go through her trash. We're going to get a handwriting sample and compare it to what's on the postcard—"

I laughed despite myself, grateful for my indefatigable friend. The whole debacle was the most confounding turn yet in my long, punishing quest for answers.

Courtney's half-joking suggestion was exactly what the old me would have done. I would have demanded a tidy resolution and stopped at nothing until I'd reached it, no matter how many dumpsters I'd have to sift through. In making the decision to "put it down," I thought I had grown past the point of wanting external validation for what happened. But the arrival of the postcard had pulled me right back into the eye of the storm.

I asked Gracie for her thoughts as we sat in her bedroom. "Why would someone go through the trouble of sending me a postcard and not signing it?" I said for the millionth time.

"Mom," Gracie said earnestly, "you've been given everything you need."

"What do you mean?" I said.

"Sometimes things are too painful to process, but whoever sent it is letting you know that you're not alone," she said. "This might be all they're ready to share right now, or maybe ever. I think you should let that be enough. Maybe she doesn't want to have a whole long conversation about it. Maybe she just needed to tell."

She was right. I could see that I had done what I always did: I pushed. The same way I had spent years pushing myself to the limit, whether it was how many miles I could run or how much I could pack into my calendar. I sought validation from outside myself when I wasn't secure within myself. This was just another example. For all the ways I had managed to "put it down," there was some part of me that still clung to the belief that someone else would validate my experience and make it all better. This curveball with Claudia had caused me to backslide. But I knew that backsliding had its own lesson to teach me.

What would it be like, I wondered, to just let go? Not to hang on tighter in this moment of discomfort but to loosen my grip—to release—to surrender to the not knowing?

All these years I had wondered: *How do I prove to others that this happened to me?* But I had tied myself in knots trying to control it all when that was just life—a series of unsolvable mysteries and unanswerable questions, invitations to let go when everything in you wants to hold on tighter. Cryptic messages from the universe, scrawled on postcards with no return address.

THE OTHER THING, THE stranger thing, was that I understood this sender, whoever they were. If there was anything I had learned about the mind, it was the way you could know something and not know it at the same time. I thought back to that day, so many years ago, with the physical therapist whom I had visited and the way she'd seen my tell. I'd backed away because I wasn't ready for the truth. I had known then, and also, I hadn't. The secret was so big I could not ignore it, and yet the size of it made it impossible to see.

I thought about my volleyball coach, Bess. This was the paradox of surviving sexual abuse, as Bess told me she herself had. Surviving abuse should have sensitized us to it, and yet the very fact of our survival made it more difficult for us to see it, in our own lives or in the lives of others. It wasn't as simple as knowing or not knowing.

If the postcard was indeed from Claudia, I knew why she would deny having sent it. By showing up in her life after so many years, I had disrupted her own denial, making hairline fractures in the glass case that kept her safe, through which the postcard had slipped. There are so many layers to awareness, the conscious and the unconscious and all the places in between.

Remembering isn't something you do just once. Remembering is a practice. It is something you have to be brave enough to do over and over again. To face the monster under your bed and to discover that there was never a monster at all but the child you once were, a child who has only been waiting for you to come back home. And then, when you forget, or blot it out because the pain is unbearable, to gather your strength and face it again. To return to this fundamental truth, no matter how many times it takes.

That was why I had needed my own child to help me remember. It was Gigi who had wept on her bed that night, asking where I was. In her voice was the cry of the little girl I had been, the little girl I myself had left behind in that middle-school bathroom all those years before, when I dissociated because the pain was too great. When she called for me, I heard the echo of my own abandoned inner child, pulling me back to where it all began.

"This all started because of you," I told her one night, sitting in her bedroom. "You knew something was off with me, and you confronted me, and that completely changed my life."

"Mom, you give me too much credit," she said. "But thanks. I am really intuitive."

AS TIME WENT ON, I found myself asking more people if I could share my story with them. I understood that it was a lot to hear, and the person listening needed to be ready to hear it. But I also understood that to tell—the thing I promised I would never do—was a gift to myself. Each time I gave myself permission to tell, I felt freer.

Sometimes, when I told people, they praised me for doing "the work," because, they said, it made me a better example to my children, a better wife to my husband, or a better friend to those closest to me. Women are always doing things so we can be better for other people. My relationships had changed for the better, but I didn't do it for anyone else. I did it for me.

There is also, I've learned, a way that people sometimes respond when I tell them about my experience. They grow tight, zipped up, locked away. "I don't think I could do anything like that," they say. "I'm too much of a control freak. And besides, I don't think I want to know. What if I don't have the space for it? What if I find out something that I can't deal with? I don't have the time to process what comes up on the other end. Why would I want to wallow in the pain?" Or the line I hear the most: "If I don't remember something, isn't there a good reason for that?" In these comments, I hear the sound of their tell—the thing that nags at them with gnawed edges, the way it did at me for so long.

Olivia laughed when I told her this. "You and I both know those are probably the people who need it the most," she said. "Just like you did."

She was visiting me and John on a summer night not unlike the one when she'd first entered my life. MDMA had recently been legalized for therapeutic use in Australia, which indicated that the rest of the Western world would likely follow in the years to come. I was wearing the bracelet Olivia had given me for my birthday a year earlier, which had become one of my most cherished possessions—a tangible link to the leap of faith I'd taken. Just like the one I'd held on her wrist during my first session, the bracelet was made of coins that I now knew dated to 1912, the year MDMA was invented.

"This medicine is going to help so many people," I said. It was funny now to think that I had been so judgmental about it.

"It already has," Olivia said. "We just haven't been able to talk about it."

I thought back to how much work I'd done in the immediate aftermath of my sessions, and how much I'd struggled with anxiety, flashbacks, and depression. I remembered how much I'd relied on John, my family, and Lauren at the time. Without them, I didn't know where I'd be.

"People are going to need resources," I said. "So if they open up the way I did, they have the space and support to sort through it slowly and integrate what happened."

"Yes, you were so lucky," Olivia said. "These sessions can be destabilizing, so it's important to remember: This medicine has to be treated with great reverence and an abundance of caution."

John had been reading about the history of psychedelics, from the indigenous peoples who first used plant medicines during ceremonial rites up through the discovery of MDMA in a laboratory. "It was never intended to be taken recreationally," he said. "The people who started using it, back in the seventies, thought of it as a tool for healing and transformation. It was first used in therapy to help patients open up emotionally."

"So what happened?" I asked. "How did it become known as a party drug?"

"Marketing," John said. "The dealer who helped make it big in America rebranded it. He called it Ecstasy because he thought it would sell better. But you know what I just learned? The medicine's first name was"—he grinned—"*Therapy*."

In my continued work with Lauren, I was learning that progress wasn't linear, that it was fine to take one step forward and two steps back, that there were still places where I wanted to control and moments when I found myself chasing an ideal of perfection—wanting to please others, to win their approval like it was another trophy I could put up on a shelf, as if that would keep me safe. But it was a relief to know that I was never going back to the way it was before— that no matter what happened, I would always know myself now.

Lauren reminded me not to give too much credit to the MDMA—that I was the one who had ultimately done the work, even if I'd had a lot of help. "This is something you did," she said. "Nobody could do it for you. It was one of your many acts of courage we could point to along this journey."

"I think all the time about that quote from Jung," I said. "We have to make the unconscious conscious, or it will direct our life and we will call it fate."

Lauren smiled. "We do," she said. "But also, Jung never said that."

"What?" I said. "Are you sure?"

"It's frequently misattributed to him," she said. "He actually said a few things along those lines, but they're all less catchy than that."

"I thought I remembered it perfectly," I said.

"Right," Lauren said. "But maybe it's not about remembering it perfectly, Amy." I looked at her. "You remembered the essential truth of it. The part of it that matters. Even if not all the specifics were exactly right. Maybe it doesn't have to be perfect. Maybe it's enough that you remembered it at all."

. . .

OVER TIME, IT BECAME easier for me to go back to Texas. There was a part of me that had always belonged there. I had just taken the long way home.

"You know when that thing happened with the milkman," my mom said once, as we were walking through the redbrick streets of Amarillo. "My dad said, 'Well, you *were* wearing short shorts.'" She shook her head. "We never talked about it. I just assumed it was my fault and tucked it away in a box somewhere."

"I'm so sorry, Mom," I said. "It wasn't your fault."

"Amy, do you ever wish you could put it all back in the box?" she asked. "That you could go back to before you knew all these horrible things?"

I didn't hesitate. "No," I said.

She looked at me, surprised by how emphatic I'd been.

"I wouldn't take any of it back," I said. "Remembering is so much better than not remembering. Telling is so much better than not telling." The sound of an ice-cream truck played somewhere in the distance. The light was bright and beautiful. "Even if facing it is hard, it's also so important. I thought of this as something I was running from. But in running from that, I was also running from the best things this life has to offer—freedom and happiness and real relationships with the people around me. You can't have light without the darkness. You have to feel all of it in order to feel any of it."

This, I suddenly realized, was why I'd needed to tell the story. Life was so dissonant in its beauties and its horrors, so full of irreconcilable truths. Telling was a way to reconcile them. Telling allowed me to process, to keep going—to live. And in that moment, I felt profound, exquisite gratitude for all I had remembered, no matter how painful it had been to face. Remembering was so hard, but now I understood why we did it—why it was worth remembering at all.

It wasn't so we could wallow in the pain. It was so we could more fully touch the joy.

DRIVING AROUND WITH MY father, we talked about the things that had changed in Texas, and the things that hadn't. "Do you remember when you used to coach me in soccer?" I asked him. "You were my first coach."

"You were always doing cartwheels," he said. "You never stopped."

"That's right," I said, laughing. "You would be trying to herd all the girls down the field, and I would be doing cartwheels, in my own world. 'Pay attention!' you'd yell across the field. 'Get in the game!' You wanted to be stern, but I could see you trying not to laugh."

"I loved it," he said. "Those were my proudest moments in life. Even though I had no idea what I was doing."

"I don't think any of us ever know what we're doing," I said. I paused. "You know, Dad, it was really confusing for me when you told me that Mom was a virgin when you married her and that you expected the same from me. Were you a virgin when you got married?"

He paused, then looked at the road instead of answering me.

"For so long I tried to do everything right," I said. "Sometimes it feels like I'm still trying to do that. Even when I got the postcard, the first thing I wanted to do was tell you, so it would validate what I'd been through. So you would believe me."

"Amy, we believed you from the beginning," he said. Through the dusty windshield, the view of the dry plains, stretching on to the horizon, was so clear. "We didn't need a postcard."

"I just worked so hard to be perfect for you," I said.

He shot me a funny look. "You never had to do anything to be perfect in my eyes," he said. "You are my daughter. You were always perfect to me."

Once more, the awareness fused together, pieces of a puzzle clicking into place.

It was so obvious. How had I missed it?

Perfect—the way every parent loves their child, not for anything they've done but just for being who they are. The way my father loved me, the way I loved my own children.

At last, I knew what perfect meant.

ON A TRIP HOME, I went for a run in Palo Duro Canyon, where I had run as a girl. The view was spectacular, and I was humbled by it, standing in the shadow of the great cliff, taking in the grandeur of my surroundings. For a moment I felt free again, like nothing could touch me. Free the way I'd been riding my banana-seat bike through the streets of Amarillo. Free as I had been as a girl doing cartwheels on the redbrick wall outside of my house.

But I understood that it was only through the telling that I had set myself free.

The landscape was orange and purple, the rock formations rugged and stark against the horizon, the sky silken blue. Atop the ridge, I saw something ambling slowly in the distance. I squinted. It looked like a longhorn. I'd heard they

AMY GRIFFIN

lived in this canyon, but I had never seen one in the wild in all the years I'd gone running there. I felt a flash of wonder. How extraordinary a sight, and how rare.

Then I squinted. It was hard to make out. Maybe it was just a shadow, or a regular old cow, out in the distance. A trick of the light, a mirage. I squinted again. I could see its form as it moved along the horizon. I could feel my body reacting to its presence—my heart beating loudly, my breath catching in my chest.

But as soon as I registered what I was seeing, it vanished. Gone again.

I would never know for sure, I thought. I'd just have to live with the uncertainty.

WHICH WAS JUST FINE.

I trusted myself.

That was enough.

I TURNED AROUND AND walked myself home.

ACKNOWLEDGMENTS

I am infinitely grateful to every person who told me that my story was worth telling.

TO THE INCREDIBLE TEAM that helped bring this book to life:

To Cait Hoyt, thank you for finding me and for telling me this story was important. You have a rare gift for simultaneously hand-holding people and their words. I am blessed to have had you by my side since day one and now to have your family in my life. Thank you to everyone at CAA—especially Ali Ehrlich for telling me I could step forward because you would be there to support me with a gentle, elegant nudge at every turn.

To Whitney Frick, thank you for telling me you wanted to help me share this story the moment we met. I know you believe in the words and that you believe in me. Thank you for teaching me how to trust myself and to allow the creative process to unfold. And oh, how I wish I had been at your wedding. Thank you also to everyone at the Dial Press and Random House—to Talia Cieslinski, Avideh Bashirrad, Debbie Aroff, Michelle Jasmine, Donna Cheng, Robert Siek, Matthew Martin, Andy Ward, Sandra Sjursen, Debbie Glasserman, and Rebecca Berlant—for treating me and my book with such thoughtful compassion.

To Sam Lansky, one of the greatest gifts of writing this book is that you are now in my life. Thank you for late-night walks with headlamps, matcha everything, and for convincing me that you would be there from the beginning to the end. You are the unicorn of truth-telling, and you make me a better me with every em dash.

To Cate, for taking on all things legal with so much heart and compassion. You once told me that you didn't know what you would do if this was your child, and you so gracefully fought for me as if I were.

My deepest gratitude to Mike Feldman, Carolyn Gluck, and everyone on the FGS team who helped me find ways to ensure other survivors could tell their stories and feel seen.

To Adam Grant, you are living proof that people appear in your life at the right moment. Thank you for shepherding me through this process, for authentically caring about me and this book, and thank you for telling me there is no need to thank you yet again for all that you have done to help share my story.

TO MY EXTRAORDINARY TEAM who kept me afloat while I wrote this book:

To Samantha Materek, the Mary Poppins of my life, thank you for selflessly standing in the wings to catch me over and over again. I hope I tell you often how grateful I am to you for all.

To Anna Doherty, the younger, faster, smarter version of me. Our partnership is truly one of a kind. I told you we could build something special, and we are doing just that together. Let's do this!

To Jackie Fernandez, thank you for being three steps ahead of me at all times and for telling me you have it all handled with grace.

To Cody Lee, my unending gratitude for keeping all the plates spinning throughout this process. I am telling you: I couldn't have done this without you.

TO THOSE WHOSE OWN stories were essential to me writing this book:

To Clara, who is wise and brilliant and who has been a mentor to me and so many girls throughout her career as an educator. Thank you for telling me every step of the way that I was meant to write this story.

To William, for telling me to put my feet on the ground and

take a deep breath. Thank you for all your wisdom. You will never know how beautifully your words landed and lifted me up in moments of deep despair.

To Bess, for being my first coach. You told me I could do anything through hard work, and I still believe that today.

To Claudia, thank you for meeting with me and for telling me I was kind. That's all I ever needed to hear from you.

TO THE FRIENDS WHO listened to me tell this story in those first weeks and months who have stood steadfastly by my side throughout:

To Courtney, my forever sidekick and doubles partner. I told you I needed you and you appeared. I am eternally grateful to you for putting your life on hold to help me reconnect with people from our past. I hope we can see more sunsets in Vega or wherever life takes us as long as you don't get carsick. I love you, Cecile.

To Rachel, who lived this story with me and whose missing tooth I would still search for today—that's how you've stood by and supported me since we were six months old. Here's to more dancing in your garage. You've always told me that you wanted me to write my book, so I guess this is it. I love you, Gayle.

To my soul sister friend, who said she would still listen to me tell this story while sitting on the front porch swing when we are eighty. Thank you for teaching me how to be a good listener. It isn't lost on me that you call every morning with coffee in hand just to let me talk. My life is brighter, funnier, and full of wonder with you in it.

To my wildly fearless friend, who holds so much for so many with endless grace, beauty, and strength. Thank you for holding me under the tree on our street for hours and for telling me my story was enough. I love you SO much, as that's what you always say to me.

To my beautiful, big sister friend, who has been a second mother to my four. You live life to the fullest. Thank you for telling me I had to join you for beach week, stuffing me in the backseat of your car all those years ago. I am with you and yours for the long haul.

To my ethereal friend, who walked with me often and told me to put my feet in the sand daily. Thank you for randomly texting me the words "I love you" over and over without ever needing a response. I could tell you were close, protecting me at all times. I love you for that and for sending me the only acceptable drip coffee maker.

To my divine upstairs neighbor friend, whose simple questions sent me looking for answers deep within. My mom wanted me to tell you that she thanks you for holding my hand when she wasn't there. Here's to many games of Ping-Pong on your terrace.

To my regal friend, who said I visited her in her dreams and that it was all going to be okay. Thank you for telling me that I don't need to retell my story to anyone ever again. It is all in the book.

To my stunning English rose friend, who calms my nervous system just by hearing your voice. Thank you for always showing up with the best advice delivered exactly at the right moment and for telling me this chapter was the beginning of something wonderful.

To my magical, trailblazer friend, who painstakingly listened as we climbed up and down a mountain in Colorado. Thank you for telling me you saw me over and over again in ways I couldn't have imagined. And thank you for showing me it is possible to build a world where kindness prevails.

To my divine friend, who left home to live where there are lemon trees but who talks like me and who says we are sort of related. I know you would be on a plane in five minutes with fresh roots, a gluten-free muffin, and a monogrammed gift if I told you I needed you.

To my talented, creative friend, who drew astonishing designs in the bathroom stalls during school lunch break. You told me it was okay to leave home and still love and be loved by those who are far away.

To my bright light of a friend, who grew up listening to Wayne Dyer tapes and who provides endless positivity. You inspire me to look for the signs and follow them. Thank you for telling and teaching me to lead with intuition.

To my truth-teller friend, who walks through life looking to help everyone in her purview and who knows that her chocolate cake makes me feel seen. Thank you for telling me about Tara Brach and for sharing every resource one could ever need in life.

To my wiser, taller, younger friend, who feels more like a little sister. Thank you for telling me not to dim my light for anyone. You have somehow found the code for a beautiful life, and it makes me smile to watch you live so fully present in your own life.

To my divinely elegant and thoughtful friend, who for twenty years has quietly helped me navigate life in New York City. You remember every milestone and constantly tell me that you are holding my hand as I move into uncharted waters.

To my magical and magnetic observer friend, who prefers to create culture rather than participate in it. You told me this book would change my life in profound ways. Now, in knowing you, I fully agree.

To my deeply kind and resilient friend, who has helped half of Manhattan in one way or another. You told me that I helped you create a new life for yourself, but it was you who literally ran toward and built the life you are living now.

To my hilarious, hardworking stunner of a friend, who has told me all the important truths of life while wearing a bathrobe. I am proud to watch you embark on this moment of being true to yourself. I'm telling you I'm here for you every step of the way.

To my superhuman friend, who races through life with deep passion and devotion all while looking quite glam. Thank you for sharing your vulnerability and for telling me I was brave in moments when the mountains felt insurmountable.

To my glowing, southern, spiritual in every sense of the word friend, who has experienced profound love and loss in her life. Thank you for telling me that amid great tragedy there is still so much joy to be felt and life to be lived.

To my brilliant walking partner, who has helped me work through so much simply standing by me step-by-step of this journey. You have told me what I am doing matters. And I've gotten to witness as you stepped into a beautiful partnership.

To my inspirational couple friends, who were going through their own journey of finding themselves again as one chapter closed and another began. Thank you for listening when I flew over to tell you my story and for always switching back into English when I am at the table so I can follow the conversation.

To my feisty, fabulous French friend, who stood with me in the days when we were told we could run a small- to medium-size country, when we fully could have taken on a large country and won with much decorum. You always fight for me and I know it!

To my gorgeous inside and out friend, who somehow manages to keep a very big life small—placing the people and the causes you care about at the center. I treasure all that we have shared and told each other in the locker room after our weekly swim practice.

To my humble, champion of a friend, who coached me through so many difficult points in the last few years. Thank you for telling me that listening is as much a skill as telling. What a blessing to stand with you as you bravely fought a difficult opponent with so much grace.

To my gentle and grounded friend, who put me back together every time I came apart. You told me what was happening in my body was physical and emotional and taught me to care for all the parts of me.

To my bold and beautiful new friend, who has felt like a very old friend in the last year. Thank you for sharing all your earned wisdom. For telling me I am worthy and for reminding me the answers are right in front of me.

To my devoted and talented friend, who sees me often through a screen. Thank you for telling me that my body was strong, not broken. I've never pretended the Wi-Fi wasn't working and gone back to bed—yet!

To my exquisite fairy friend, who helped me find clarity with movement and music. Thank you for never telling me anything,

rather you showed me how the body can let go of something difficult and turn it into something beautiful. And now it is your turn.

To my talented and always humble friend, for making me feel
seen through your lens. Your ability to capture humanity in an
image is something that I greatly admire. I want to tell you that you
deserve the beautiful life that you have fought for and are living.

To my effortlessly fabulous, superchic friend, who could simply sit with me on the floor of my closet and make me feel seen.
Thank you for telling me to go out into the world in full color and
do my thing with grace and style.

To my coach and biggest cheerleader friend, for every swim,
bike, and run. You always told me to rest and to give myself grace
as I had done the training and was ready. I think your words are
finally resonating as I publish this book.

To all my volleyball teammates, who taught me how to work
together for the greater good of the whole. Thank you for telling
me I was a leader.

And to the friend whose texts always popped up at just the
right moment. You know who you are, and I am telling you, I am
forever grateful.

TO THE WOMEN WHOSE work in the mental health space is
poised to transform the world:

To Lauren, your impressive credentials are no match for the
expansiveness of your heart. It isn't what you've told me that has
transformed my life but what you haven't said as you've let me
come to it on my own. Thank you for teaching me how to fully
trust in myself, and how to walk again.

To Olivia, the Divine Feminine, the light you cast in this world
made me feel secure enough to chart this course. You've held my
hand through the darkest of moments and told me in the aftermath that I would one day soar. You heard my words first, and I am
eternally grateful to you for listening.

To my parents, for their authentic, perfect love. In so many ways you not only told me but showed me that you believed every word. I can only hope to parent my children the way you have parented me through these last few years.

Mom, you have lived every single word of this book with me in real time. I have felt your limitless support every day of my life.

Dad, you consistently put our family above all else and at the same time built an extraordinary business of which we are all proud.

To my stunning-in-every-way sister, Lizzie, for telling me it was okay to step away while you waited for me with loving patience. You are everything in this life that I have at times run from. You have the grace of our mom, the patience of an angel, and an occasional wild streak that must come from Grammy.

To my brothers, Jeff and Andrew, whom I love dearly and know will tell their children my story and be proud of me for writing this book. Thank you both for all that you do to further build and support the family business started by our grandmother and for all that you do for our local community.

To my boys, Jack and Julian, the bookends of our family, for telling me I was doing something important in writing this book not only for women but also for men.

To my girls, Gracie and Gigi, for helping me face my truth. You are my greatest teachers, and I love you dearly. I will forever tell you both how much you inspire me.

To John, there are no words. Your actions speak louder than words. I don't have to tell you anything. You already know, I love you.

To Alice, Jeannine, and Novie, for telling me I was special. I tried so hard to believe them. I know they are with me on this journey, and I hope these words make them proud.

And finally, to my almost ninety-seven-year-old Grampy, who I haven't told my story to but love without limit. He's lived through the Dust Bowl, the Great Depression, and countless wars. If there is anyone who has taught me to survive, it is you.

RESOURCES

Confronting memories of childhood abuse, particularly those suppressed by the conscious mind, is a difficult and disruptive process. I was extraordinarily fortunate that I had access to the resources, support, and relationships to help navigate my new reality.

There is no one-size-fits-all approach to processing complex trauma; I learned what worked for me through a process of experimentation and discovery. This resource guide, while by no means comprehensive, includes many of the tools and additional reading materials that I found helpful in my own recovery, as well as organizations that are doing critical work to help survivors.

To access this resource guide, please visit www.thetellbook .com/resources.

As extraordinary as these resources are, the single most vital tool that I discovered on my journey was my ability to tell: to share my story and forge connections with those who could listen. May this book inspire you to share your own story—remembering that, in the telling, we unbind the shame and discover new hope.

ABOUT THE AUTHOR

Amy Griffin lives in New York City with her husband, John, and their four children. She is the founder of G9 Ventures, an early-stage investment firm.

thetellbook.com
Instagram: @amygriffin

Books Driven by the Heart

Sign up for our newsletter
and find more you'll love:

thedialpress.com

Amy Griffin lives in New York City with her husband, John, and their four children. She is the founder of G9 Ventures, an early-stage investment firm.

thetellbook.com
Instagram: @amygriffin

Books Driven by the Heart

Sign up for our newsletter and find more you'll love:

thedialpress.com

@THEDIALPRESS

@THEDIALPRESS